THE Fertility CODE

DEDICATION

To Faye, Alison, Grace, Holly, Rory and Dylan. You remind me what this book is all about and bless my life each and every day.

To Yvonne, for being you … and such an absolute inspiration.

And to Joe, thank you for being a true friend and great brother.

THE Fertility CODE

Dermot O'Connor

First published in 2012 by Y Books
Lucan, Co. Dublin, Ireland
Tel/fax: +353 1 6217992
publishing@ybooks.ie
www.ybooks.ie

Paperback	ISBN: 978-1-908023-39-1
Ebook – Mobi format	ISBN: 978-1-908023-40-7
Ebook – epub format	ISBN: 978-1-908023-41-4

A CIP catalogue record for this book is available from the British Library.

Cover design by Graham Thew Design
Cover images: www.istockphoto.com

CONTENTS

ACKNOWLEDGEMENTS

This book could not have happened without the help and support of many people to whom I would like to extend my sincerest appreciation.

A special thank you to Paul McKenna. Without his support this book would never have been written.

I am very grateful to Chenile Keogh and Robert Doran. It has been an absolute pleasure to work with Y Books and I very much appreciate their support throughout this project.

Sincere thanks to Dr David Walsh, to the team at Sims IVF Clinic and especially to Ann Bracken for her valuable contribution to this book.

Finally my thanks go to my patients, who have embraced and illuminated many of the principles of this book. Their inspiring stories have revealed the true power of the Fertility Code.

THE
Fertility CODE
Introduction

"A baby will make love stronger, days shorter, nights longer, bankroll smaller, home happier, clothes shabbier, the past forgotten, and the future worth living for"

Anonymous

YOU'RE NOT ALONE

Having a baby is probably the most significant thing you will achieve in your lifetime. Across cultures, continents and generations, the birth of a baby is something that elevates and unites us and provides our single clearest glimpse into the divine. It is a tragedy then that for many couples the blessing of reproduction becomes almost a curse as they try and try, without success, to conceive a child together.

It is estimated that one in six couples in the UK and Ireland will face fertility challenges. This represents over four million people and the number has been on the rise in recent decades.

You are most likely reading this book because you hope to have a baby and have recently started trying to conceive, or you may have been trying for quite some time, without success. You may also have decided to seek the support of a fertility clinic to medically assist your efforts to achieve pregnancy. Whatever the case, you certainly want to know what you can do for yourself to increase your chances of having a baby. You are not alone on this journey; there are millions of others on the same road, encountering the same challenges you are dealing with.

Having a baby is part and parcel of most people's life plans. Finding a partner, settling down and buying a home are all steps towards that goal of starting a family. We embark on this journey, like millions of our ancestors who followed a similar path. It is an innate impulse to want to produce offspring. Since the dawning of humanity all of your direct ancestors have been fertile. Therefore for many of us there is an assumption that we will be no different.

People come to my clinic for a variety of reasons, including a whole host of medical complaints. But it is my work with couples who wish to start a family that I find the most rewarding. These couples are probably the most highly motivated of all of my clients, beyond even those facing life-challenging illnesses. The joy that success brings when couples bring home their healthy baby is incomparable.

I believe that taking control of your fertility is crucial to the process of having a baby. The Fertility Code is all about empowering you to take charge of your fertility and this book will support and guide you on that voyage, taking a multidimensional approach by working at psychological, emotional, nutritional, physical and medical levels.

The Fertility Code is, I believe, worthwhile for all couples hoping to have a baby. This book will provide you with many answers, whether you are just starting out on your journey or you are a battle-weary veteran. You may have even been told that you are never likely to have a baby. I believe that just as there are always things you can do to improve your health, there are also always things you can do to optimise your fertility.

The realisation that you can influence your fertility is a very potent one for couples. Of course there will be situations where medical and physical obstacles may stand in your way, but even in these cases there are choices and opportunities. When you understand that you have options, it provides both hope and motivation, which will help you take positive steps towards greater fertility.

When we think about someone attending a fertility clinic, we typically imagine a woman. But it obviously takes two people to conceive a baby, and if there are problems, 50 per cent of the time this is to do with the man. The Fertility Code therefore seeks to enhance fertility for both men and women.

♀♂

Why the Fertility Code?

The Fertility Code is designed to prepare you for healthy conception and successful pregnancy. Using powerful and proven strategies, you will prime your body to become as fertile as possible. Detailed step-by-step instructions will show you how to implement these strategies. For many couples, this will be all that is required in order to naturally achieve a healthy pregnancy in as little as three months. Countless couples have come to my clinic having been on an unproductive fertility journey for many years and have conceived within just a few weeks of implementing the Fertility Code.

Some couples may need to continue to seek medical help, but they will do so in the knowledge that they are doing everything possible to support this process. The combination of modern medical reproductive treatment and taking steps to naturally enhance your fertility is very powerful and effective. Whatever your situation, by following the Fertility Code, you can be certain that you are increasing your chances of success.

The Fertility Code follows the integrated approach successfully taken by patients at our clinics. Our plan combines the latest understandings from Western reproductive medicine with the age old wisdom of Eastern medicine. This is a happy and successful marriage that has proven a most effective approach in treating fertility across the globe. Within the laboratory environment of the fertility clinic it has been scientifically established that when Western medical fertility treatment is combined with Eastern and mind/body medicine techniques such as acupuncture and mindfulness, the conception success rates are approximately 65 per cent higher. This is why the most farsighted fertility clinics now offer medical acupuncture and mind/body programmes as part of their normal service. Not to do so would in fact be turning a blind eye to an overwhelming amount of scientific evidence.

Whilst the Fertility Code is designed to naturally enhance your reproductive health, it also acknowledges that it makes sense to draw upon the considerable wisdom and support of the medical profession. So although Eastern medicine and mind/body approaches play a significant role in addressing reproductive issues at our clinics, they work in combination with the knowledge of Western medical principles. This combination of influences from East and West ensures that our clients get the very best of both worlds.

♀♂

Case study – Jane and Will

For Jane and Will it seemed that fertility problems would torment them for ever. When Jane and Will first came to my clinic, they were both in their early thirties and had been trying to have a child together for four years. At first they had been unconcerned that months went by without success, but after the first year of trying, anxiety began to creep in. Jane noticed that more and more of her friends were having babies. Work colleagues returning from maternity leave would inevitably show off photos of their children, and Jane was finding it increasingly difficult to hide her distress. The problem was taking its toll on Jane and Will's relationship and it seemed to them that there was a hole that only a baby could fill.

When they were both aged thirty, Jane and Will finally went to their GP to find out what the problem was. Their GP was understanding and referred the couple for a battery of tests. At this time they began to feel hopeful once more. At last they would get to the root of the problem and hopefully take steps to address it and be able to bring a child into the world together.

The test results finally came in – and they were devastating. 'In a way I would have preferred if the tests had shown that one of us was unwell, or had identified a specific problem,' Will told me. Instead the results came back negative; there was no problem that the doctors could identify. 'Our fertility problem was just unexplained – a mystery.'

It was at this point that Jane and Will came to see me, and I was able to help them to stand back and take a fresh, optimistic look at their fertility challenge. During the initial consultation with Jane, when I asked what her general health was like, she answered that it was fine and there were no real problems.

However, on closer inspection there were numerous subtle signs that all was not as well as it could be. There was nothing so severe that it merited going to the doctor. However, the combination of a variety of symptoms gave a strong indication that there were deficiencies that needed to be addressed in order to improve their chances of having a baby.

Using the Fertility Code, the couple were able to optimise their health and fertility and they overcome the obstacles in their path. Today, Jane and Will are proud parents of two happy and healthy children.

♀♂

There is no shortage of people who are ready to offer fertility advice and homespun wisdom, whether it's your friends, family or an afternoon TV show. It seems that every second magazine has suggestions for improving your fertility. Because there is so much information out there, it can become overwhelming for many couples and often they become confused about which path they should follow. The Fertility Code will focus your mind by giving you a full and comprehensive understanding of your health, lifestyle and fertility. It will guide you to making the most sensible and reasoned choices.

Fertility in the modern world

The advent of the technological age promised to give us more leisure time. We were told that with much less effort we would be able to achieve the same or even greater productivity, leaving us with far more time for ourselves. What has transpired couldn't be further from this ideal. We are now expected to cram more than ever into our day. Working lunches, being contactable via mobile phone 24/7 and operating across multiple time zones have now become the norm. Just to keep up, the average couple often postpones starting a family until they are better established in their careers, and for many this means waiting until later in life. For most of humanity's existence on this planet life expectancy was no greater than forty years. The phenomenon of wanting to conceive in later adulthood is a very modern one. Biologically we have not yet evolved to cope with this modern trend. In fact, a woman's fertility starts to decline from her early twenties and drops sharply in her thirties and beyond. Many couples make the conception of their child part of their 'project plan'. In an effort to meet the project deadlines they are prepared to undergo all sorts of treatments, when really what they need to do first is take a step back and look at the bigger picture.

♀♂

MY STORY AND THE DEVELOPMENT OF THE FERTILITY CODE

In 1998 I was a successful executive travelling the globe and working all hours, when suddenly I was struck by severe vertigo, slurred speech and numbness all over my body. After extensive medical tests, including an MRI scan and a lumbar puncture, my neurologist gave me the shocking diagnosis – I had a severe and aggressive form of multiple sclerosis (MS) that was likely to see me confined to a wheelchair within twelve to twenty-four months. This news was absolutely devastating, as in one fell swoop my dreams for the future were swept away and I was advised to prepare myself mentally for a 'managed decline' – the clinical euphemism for an inexorable slide into dependency, disease and death.

At first I accepted my fate with grave despair. The more I educated myself about the hardships MS could inflict, the more I noticed the condition seep into every fibre of my body, and it seemed to sap the very life-blood from my being.

However, after going through the deepest despair, I drew on resources within myself to harness the power of my subconscious mind, to move myself mentally towards hope. I embarked on a journey that would take me around the world to train with some of the leading figures in the areas of mind/body medicine, nutrition and various branches of Eastern medicine. In my mind's eye I created a positive vision of health and vitality, and with the help of the extensive lifestyle changes I had made, I moved towards this vision with complete confidence. By 2006 I was symptom free and in fantastic health, and I published my first book, *The Healing Code*, in which I told my story and detailed my approach to the treatment of and recovery from serious health issues such as heart disease, cancer and multiple sclerosis. My belief is that your body is constantly trying to heal itself of illnesses such as type 2 diabetes, and that this task can be supported by nutrition and detoxification. This was met with scepticism in some quarters. But in 2011 I was delighted when a Newcastle University team 'discovered' that type 2 diabetes can be reversed by a diet which bore many of the hallmarks of the Healing Code Nutrition Plan.

Generally speaking, however, the medical profession has supported my approach. In 2006 when I was interviewed on BBC's *The Heaven and Earth Show*, Dr Mark Hamilton was invited to offer a medical, and perhaps sceptical, view of my approach. I was delighted when he said that almost every doctor he knew would be happy if people read and followed *The Healing Code*. He believed that people need to take responsibility for their health as well as seeking the proper medical attention. We were in complete agreement.

Whilst researching my second book, *The Immortality Code*, which outlined my approach to achieving healthy longevity, I visited the advanced diagnostic clinic, Cenegenics, in South Carolina, USA. My test results at the clinic established that I was one of the fittest and healthiest people that they had ever assessed. Later in 2008 I was honoured to be acknowledged by my peers when I was elected as Chairman of The Acupuncture Council of Ireland. I had gone from experiencing first-hand the benefits of Eastern medicine in 1998 as part of my recovery to representing the largest Eastern medicine organisation in Ireland.

Due to the success of my books I was able to reach out to people from all over the world who had used my system to help them recover from a variety of challenging illnesses. My Healing Code Clinics became a source of respite for thousands of people seeking to harness my approach in dealing with health challenges. Although I encountered many conditions at my clinics, there was one health issue that accounted for the majority of my clients – fertility.

In Eastern medicine the approach to treating fertility is really quite simple and logical: in order to be as fertile as possible, a couple should be as healthy as possible. Just as the soil in a garden needs to be healthy for flowers to grow, the physical and mental well-being of a couple should be maximised in order to improve the chances of having a healthy baby. I was able to adapt the principles of the Healing Code and apply these to support couples in their goal of having a baby. Very soon this approach started to result in considerable success for many couples and word spread that my Healing Code Clinic was a place to visit for any couple encountering fertility problems. And so the Fertility Code was born.

♀♂

WHAT THE FERTILITY CODE WILL DO FOR YOU

The Fertility Code is designed to prepare your and your partner's bodies for healthy conception and pregnancy. The strategies of the Fertility Code will boost your sense of well-being and in the process prime you to achieve what nature intended. The basic laws of natural selection state that the healthiest of the species will also be the most successful at reproducing. Therefore the better you feel and the healthier you are, the more likely it is that you will have a healthy baby.

If you decide to use assisted reproductive technologies, the Fertility Code will act as a foundation to support your body for fertility treatment, increasing the chances of success as well as the ease with which it can be achieved. Couples who use the advanced technologies of the modern fertility clinic still need to ensure that their bodies are physically primed to be receptive to medical intervention. As advanced as it is, the process still relies on nature and medicine working together in harmony.

This book will give you and your partner a complete plan of action that will help to maximise your chances of having a healthy baby. It will help you:

℔ Balance your hormone levels

- ♘ Regulate your menstrual cycle

- ♘ Restore and enhance your ovulation cycle

- ♘ Protect against repeated and early miscarriages

- ♘ Improve sperm count and sperm motility

- ♘ Attain optimum nutrition and supplementation for conception.

- ♘ De-stress your mind and body

- ♘ Remove harmful toxins that diminish fertility

- ♘ Deal with medical problems that present a physical obstacle to conception

- ♘ Give birth to a healthy baby!

♀ ♂

HOW THIS BOOK IS STRUCTURED

To help you understand and implement the principles of the Fertility Code, I have organised this book into seven key chapters. Successfully conceiving, going full-term with your pregnancy and delivering a healthy baby may seem like a long and difficult journey, but with the correct map you can find your way with a sure footing.

In chapter one we will look at the basic understanding of male and female fertility and at what exactly is involved in getting pregnant naturally. Whilst it is assumed that you know about the birds and bees, it is surprising how confused many people are about the biology of reproduction and getting pregnant. There are crucial elements that are helpful for you to understand if you wish to conceive. We will examine the male and female reproductive systems with particular emphasis on how to establish when a couple is at their most fertile.

In chapters two and three we will look at the psychology of fertility. It has been recognised by gynaecologists that stress has a significant impact on fertility. For many couples the process of trying to conceive can in itself become incredibly stressful. We will look at how your brain and emotions affect your body and detail proven methods to develop an increased sense of calm and tranquillity as you embark on your fertility journey.

Chinese medicine understands that where the mind goes the body will follow. In these chapters we will also look at ways to support the mind/body connection to maximise fertility at optimum times within your cycle. We will examine powerful mental techniques that have been used for centuries to actively increase the potential for conception.

In chapter four we will examine what is perhaps the most important aspect of your lifestyle – nutrition. This is an area that is completely within your control, and some of the latest research has discovered that your diet has a much greater impact on your fertility than previously thought. There are many diet books on the market that deal with weight loss, most detailing some quirky new approach in order to be different. The Fertility Code Nutrition Plan is different in that it uses good old common sense, and whilst it will help you to lose weight if that is what you need to do, its main focus is on actively increasing your chances of conception.

In chapter five you will take control of the habits, behaviours and toxins that are compromising, and often damaging, your fertility. I will deliver an effective strategy that will help you conquer unhelpful dietary and environmental pollutants, including tobacco, alcohol and other toxins that are proven to have a negative impact on you and your partner's ability to have a baby.

In chapter six you will learn about exercise and achieving your ideal body weight. Exercise has a huge effect on the body and it also plays a role in fertility. When exercising to increase fertility, it is important for both men and women to get the balance right. Many people mistakenly think that the more exercise you do the healthier and more fertile you become. This is not correct. Too much exercise and your fertility levels can drop greatly, especially if you're underweight. On the flip side, too little or no exercise can lower your chances of conceiving, especially if you're overweight. The goal is to find a happy medium that keeps your fertility levels high, and your body healthy.

Chapter seven concentrates on some of the medical issues that can stand in the way of conceiving and how you can overcome them.

How soon will it start working?

In my clinics I have met hundreds of people who have experienced fertility challenges. I meet people at every stage of the journey to starting a family. In Chinese medicine they say that the best time to treat a person is the year before they are born. In other words, Chinese medicine fully recognises the importance of both parents being healthy and contented before a child is even conceived. During my training I was often warned to be careful when treating young women because in the process of helping someone to improve their health and well-being you invariably make them more fertile, and hence much more susceptible to becoming pregnant. This 'danger' has of course become a great advantage to many of my clients and the benefits of a holistic approach to fertility have been proven over and over again.

The Fertility Code is designed as a three-month programme but the good news is that you should start to experience a positive effect on your fertility from the outset. Attentive and on-going adherence to the programme may rapidly result in pregnancy, but if not, the feeling of improved health, greater self-awareness and mental well-being will be an undoubted advantage in achieving a healthy pregnancy, and something you'll want to sustain well after your baby is born.

How to read this book

"If I hear I forget; if I see I remember; if I do I make it my own"
Chinese proverb

This book is structured to guide you and your partner in a logical and clear manner on your path to having a baby. Throughout the sections of the book you will be called on to make decisions, perform tasks and take action. I encourage both you and your partner to seize the moment and respond immediately on these occasions. The Fertility Code works, but it only works when you put the programme into action.

You might discover that some principles of the Fertility Code are already familiar to you. That's great. But do ask yourself, 'Am I currently implementing these principles?' If not, make a firm commitment to put them into action – now!

I recognise that any lifestyle changes require mental fortitude. It is for this reason that an early element of the programme is the Fertile Mind which will help ensure that you are mentally prepared for this journey.

If you find yourself resisting some of the Fertility Code steps, or if some of the exercises don't make immediate sense to you, or if you find yourself completing exercises in your head when they should be written down, bear in mind that most resistance occurs when the need for change is greatest. Embrace the change with the determination and the confidence that you are moving forward towards your ultimate objective.

So let us begin our journey.

♀♂

THE
Basics OF
Fertility

"Life is a flame that is always burning itself out, but it catches fire again every time a child is born"

George Bernard Shaw

INTRODUCTION

Fertility issues are far more common than many people think. When you are yearning to start a family it might seem that everyone around you is expecting or having babies. However, the truth is that conceiving can be difficult. As many as one in three of us will encounter stress and anxiety related to fertility. Some of this stress and anxiety can be alleviated if we gain a deeper understanding of fertility and conception. Let's start with a quick reminder of some of the basics of biology, which may help to dispel some common myths about fertility.

♀ ♂

WHY ISN'T IT HAPPENING FOR US?

Life starts with a sequence of two events. First of all an active sperm finds its way into a mature egg. Then this fertilised egg settles into the lining of the uterus and begins to develop.

This all sounds quite simple, but within this process are many other mini steps influenced by a sequence of carefully timed hormone releases that are needed to make the sperm active and the egg mature. For conception to occur there has to be a perfectly coordinated assembly of hormones, physiology and environmental factors.

A fertile and perfectly healthy couple at prime reproductive age (i.e. in their mid twenties) has about a one in four chance of conceiving each month if they are actively trying to become pregnant. Just about half of couples attain pregnancy within six months. Only when we extend this period to two years will approximately 90 per cent of these couples attain pregnancy. So everything might be functioning fine, but after six months of trying, many perfectly fertile couples will become stressed and anxious even though there is no physical reason why they shouldn't conceive. Of course when stress and anxiety become a factor, you are dealing with something that has a negative impact on fertility, which we will discuss further later.

So how can you tell if there actually is something wrong? I would suggest that couples who are aged thirty-five or under seek medical advice if they have not attained pregnancy after twelve months of regular unprotected sex. For those over thirty-five it makes sense to seek this advice sooner, and I would recommend that medical fertility analysis and advice should be sought after four to six months.

It is certainly true that age is a factor when hoping to conceive, and while less than 10 per cent of couples in their early twenties will have fertility issues, this rises to 30 per cent for couples in their early forties. Pressure on couples to develop their careers before starting a family means that more and more people are encountering fertility issues related to their age. However, it's worth bearing in mind that this statistic also means that 70 per cent of couples in their early forties will not have issues with fertility. It is only when we consider those over forty-five that we see fertility problems affecting over 50 per cent of couples.

Age, however, is not the only factor and I would contend that an equally important factor is good health. Good health can be evaluated in a number of ways and takes into account a variety of elements such as diet, lifestyle and stress, both environmental and occupational. Whilst we cannot turn back our chronological age we can almost entirely control these other important elements and thereby boost our chances of conceiving a healthy baby. Before exploring how the Fertility Code can optimise your fertility, let's set the stage with a quick review of the main things that must happen for conception to occur.

Most people know some of the basics of reproductive health,

but having a complete understanding is important if you want to increase your chances of a successful pregnancy. Let us look first of all at the female reproductive system.

♀ ♂

THE FEMALE REPRODUCTIVE SYSTEM

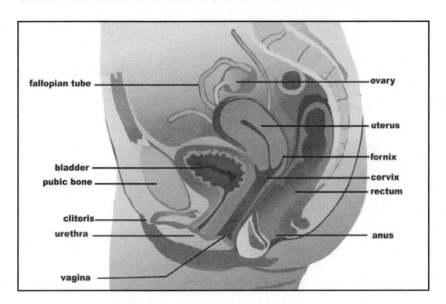

Parts of the female reproductive system

The female reproductive system carries out several functions. It produces the egg cells necessary for reproduction, which are called the ova or oocytes. It then transports the ova to the site of fertilisation. Conception, when the egg is fertilised by a sperm, usually occurs in the fallopian tubes, and the next stage of the process is for the fertilised egg to implant itself in the walls of the uterus. These are the initial stages of pregnancy. If fertilisation and/or implantation do not take place, menstruation occurs, which is the monthly shedding of the uterine lining. The female reproductive system also produces the sex hormones that maintain the reproductive cycle.

The female reproductive system includes parts both inside and outside the body. The external female reproductive structures enable sperm to enter the body and also protect the internal genital organs from infections.

The main female reproductive structures include:

℔ Labia majora – Literally translated as 'large lips', these protect the other external reproductive organs. The labia majora are relatively large and fleshy and contain sweat and oil-secreting glands.

℔ Labia minora – Literally translated as 'small lips', these lie just inside the labia majora, and surround the openings to the vagina and urethra.

℔ Clitoris – The clitoris is where the two labia minora meet. It is a small, sensitive protrusion that is comparable to the male penis. The clitoris is covered by a fold of skin called the prepuce. Like the penis, the clitoris is very sensitive to stimulation.

℔ Vagina – The vagina is a canal that joins the cervix (the lower part of the uterus) to the outside of the body. This is also known as the birth canal.

℔ Uterus – The uterus, also known as the womb, is a hollow, pear-shaped organ that is home to a developing baby. The uterus has two parts: the cervix, which is at the lower part and opens into the vagina, and the main body of the uterus, which is called the corpus. The corpus can expand to accommodate a developing baby. A passage through the cervix allows sperm to enter and menstrual blood to exit.

℔ Ovaries – The ovaries are small, oval glands located on either side of the uterus. The ovaries produce eggs and hormones.

℔ Fallopian tubes – These are the narrow tubes that are attached to the upper part of the uterus and serve as passages for the ova (egg cells) to travel from the ovaries to the uterus. Conception normally occurs in the fallopian tubes and then the fertilised egg moves to the uterus, where it implants into the lining of the uterus walls.

When a girl is born she is estimated to have between 500,000 and two million immature eggs divided between tiny ovaries. She will not make any new eggs during her lifetime. By the onset of puberty, this number has already dropped to between 300,000 and 400,000. During her menstruating years, a woman will release on average about 400 eggs. Although each menstrual cycle will usually see the ovaries releasing one egg, a woman's body actually prepares about twenty immature eggs each month for release. However, usually only one egg will be dominant and this is the egg that is released at ovulation. During each month approximately 1,000 eggs will die and this phenomenon happens regardless of any hormone production, pregnancies, nutritional supplements or health and lifestyle issues. When the woman finally runs out of her supply of eggs, the ovaries cease to produce oestrogen and she will begin menopause.

A woman's reproductive years therefore by definition begin at puberty when she starts menstruating and end when she enters menopause, usually between the ages of forty-five and fifty. Whilst the average length of a menstrual cycle is twenty-eight days, it is very common for a cycle to last anywhere between twenty-one and thirty-five days. Most women on average have menstrual flow for three to five days but it is also very common to menstruate for as long as seven days.

THE MENSTRUAL CYCLE

The first weeks

What determines your fertility begins in the brain, not in the reproductive organs. An area of the brain called the hypothalamus regulates many functions of the body, like our desire to eat, drink, sleep, have sex, and other hormonal or endocrine functions that regulate fertility.

The first day of a woman's period is the beginning of the menstrual cycle. Oestrogen levels are at their lowest at this time and this sends a signal to your brain to release follicle stimulating hormone releasing factor (FSH-RF). The pituitary gland then starts releasing follicle stimulating hormone (FSH). As more FSH is produced, usually between fifteen and twenty egg follicles begin to mature. However, most of the FSH will be attracted to just one of these egg follicles and it will then produce oestradiol, which is the major oestrogen and main sex hormone in a woman's body. The pituitary gland then receives the signal to taper off the production of FSH and as it does so the weaker egg follicles begin to die off.

When oestrogen production increases, the uterine lining starts to thicken and the cervical mucus becomes more fluid and slippery – perfect for sperm to move in.

Ovulation

Oestrogen levels rise steadily from the beginning of the menstrual cycle. About thirty-six hours before ovulation, oestrogen levels peak, stimulating the pituitary gland to release a surge of luteinising hormone (LH). When the follicle releases the egg, the fallopian tubes collect it and it then travels down towards the uterus. This process is called ovulation.

When ovulation has happened, the follicle that had been holding the egg will shrink and begin to gather a fatty substance, or lipid, and then produce progesterone. As the follicle secretes more progesterone, the uterine lining readies itself for implantation of a fertilised egg.

When the egg is released, there is approximately a twenty-four-hour window during which the sperm can fertilise it. However, the actual fertile window is longer than this because the sperm may already be present from intercourse that has taken place in the days immediately preceding ovulation.

Menstruation

If an egg has been successfully fertilised and implants into the uterine lining, the woman's body will begin to secrete another hormone: human chorionic gonadotropin (hCG). This hormone helps to maintain the production of oestrogen and progesterone for the remainder of the pregnancy.

If an egg is not fertilised, it will continue its journey and will be expelled from the body along with the endometrial lining. This is of course what is called a period. Menstruation may also occur if an egg has been fertilised but it has not implanted in the uterine lining. If this has happened the fertilised egg will be expelled together with the endometrium during the period. When no pregnancy occurs during a cycle, the corpus luteum – the follicle that has released the egg – dries up and hormone levels begin to fall. As these hormone levels drop, the hypothalamus is stimulated to start producing gonadotropin releasing hormone (GnRH), which signals to the pituitary gland to start secreting FSH again, and so the menstrual cycle continues.

Menstrual cycle FAQs

Does ovulation always take place on the fourteenth day after your period starts?

The day of ovulation can differ from woman to woman and for each woman can differ from month to month. The fourteenth-day idea seems to come simply from taking the average cycle length of twenty-eight days and dividing this in half. However, this is not an accurate way to time ovulation as many women do not ovulate on the fourteenth day of their cycle. Ovulation generally occurs somewhere between day ten and day nineteen, or twelve to sixteen days before the next period is due. Knowing when ovulation occurs is important if you want to increase the likelihood of conception.

How long is the fertility window during the ovulation phase?

During the ovulation phase, an egg is available to be fertilised for about twelve to twenty-four hours. However, as sperm can survive in the woman's body for between three to five days, it can be ready on the day the egg is released. The fertility window is therefore considered to be between five and six days. We will discuss the importance of this fertility window later in this chapter.

Can you ovulate when you are having your period?

For women with regular menstrual cycles, ovulating during a period is highly unlikely. Some women have very irregular cycles and can occasionally ovulate during a period or what is believed to be a period (it often isn't). However, because sperm can live in the body for three to five days, pregnancy can occur from intercourse that takes place during a period, but in this instance ovulation will have occurred shortly after your period.

Can I ovulate right after my period?

If you have a short cycle of, say, twenty-one days from the start of one period to the beginning of another and you menstruate for seven days, then yes, you could ovulate immediately after your period. This is because we know ovulation can occur twelve to sixteen days before your next period begins, and in the example above this could mean you would ovulate just after your period.

What are signs that you are ovulating?

There are a few signs of ovulation but many women may only notice one or two of these, if any.

- ✺ Changes in cervical fluid
- ✺ Changes in cervical position and cervical firmness
- ✺ Brief twinges or aches that are usually felt on one side of the abdomen
- ✺ Light spotting
- ✺ Increased sex drive
- ✺ Breast tenderness
- ✺ Abdominal bloating
- ✺ Heightened senses

Can ovulation occur without the stretchy white cervical fluid being present?

Ovulation can take place even if the stretchy egg-white-like fluid that we assume accompanies ovulation is not obvious. Different women can experience cervical fluid in different ways, but ovulation is assumed to take place on the day a woman has the greatest amount of wet cervical fluid.

Many women can experience ovulation fluid for a few days prior to ovulation and can also have it after ovulation has finished. When women are observing their fluid to determine ovulation, they are looking for the twelve- to twenty-four-hour period that they had the greatest amount of fluid. That is the time that an egg is available for fertilisation. However, because semen can survive for up to five days inside a woman's body, intercourse that happens on the few days before this may also result in pregnancy.

If an ovulation predictor test kit shows a positive result, does that mean I am definitely ovulating?

Ovulation predictor kits determine whether higher levels of LH are present. The LH rises right before ovulation occurs. The kits are designed to detect whether you're going to ovulate, but they cannot be sure of this.

Women may have a high level of LH if they have certain conditions such as polycystic ovaries, premature ovarian failure (POF), or are experiencing perimenopause. Any of these conditions could result in a false positive result on an ovulation predictor test.

Can ovulation occur more than once during each cycle?

Ovulation cannot occur more than once during each cycle, therefore a woman can only get pregnant once during a cycle. However, two or more eggs can be released in a single cycle. When two eggs are fertilised during one twenty-four-hour period this can result in the birth of fraternal twins. It is estimated that this occurs in as many as 5 to 10 per cent of all cycles but does not result in that many twins due to partial miscarriage, which often goes undetected.

Can ovulation occur without having a period?

Because a woman releases an egg twelve to sixteen days before her expected period, it is possible to ovulate and get pregnant without a period happening. A woman may not have been menstruating due to certain conditions such as low body-weight, breastfeeding, etc. but can still ovulate at any point. When trying to conceive, this absence of periods makes it more difficult to time ovulation.

Can I have a period and still not have ovulated?

Having a period will not always mean that ovulation has occurred. Some women may have what is called an anovulatory cycle where they can experience some bleeding even though ovulation has not taken place. This could be mistaken for a period, but it isn't actually a true period. This bleeding may be due to either a build-up in the uterine lining that can no longer sustain itself or because of a drop in oestrogen levels.

HORMONES

There are five main hormones involved in the menstrual cycle: oestrogen, progesterone, gonadotropin releasing hormone (GnRH), follicle stimulating hormone (FSH) and luteinising hormone (LH).

Oestrogen – Although oestrogen is thought of as a single hormone, there are in fact different forms of oestrogen produced by the female body. The two main oestrogens involved in the menstrual cycle are oestradiol and androgen. Oestradiol thickens the endometrial lining along with making vaginal and cervical mucus more receptive to sperm. Androgen, on the other hand, does not begin as oestrogen. The ovaries convert androgen into extra oestrogen. This increase in oestrogen helps to remove the immature egg follicles.

Progesterone – This hormone is produced by the follicle from which the mature egg has been released. Progesterone helps prepare the endometrial lining for implantation if an egg is fertilised during the cycle. Progesterone also stops the egg follicles from developing any further.

Gonadotopin releasing hormone (GnRH) – This hormone is produced by the hypothalamus in the brain. GnRH controls the production of and levels of oestrogen in the body. Towards the end of your cycle, your oestrogen levels bottom out and the GnRH is notified to begin producing oestrogen all over again. However, when your body starts secreting high levels of progesterone, GnRH is no longer produced.

Follicle stimulating hormone (FSH) – This hormone helps to stimulate egg follicles, thereby aiding the maturation of the eggs and increasing the production of oestradiol. FSH is secreted by the pituitary gland, which is stimulated by the hypothalamus' production of GnRH.

Luteinising hormone (LH) – This hormone is also produced by the pituitary gland in response to your body's production of GnRH. LH works with the egg follicles to produce androgen.

THE MALE REPRODUCTIVE SYSTEM

The purpose of the male reproductive system is to perform the following functions:

- ✑ To produce, maintain, and transport sperm (the male reproductive cells) and protective fluid (semen)

- ✑ To discharge sperm inside the female reproductive tract during sex

🐾 To produce and secrete the male sex hormones that are responsible for maintaining the male reproductive system

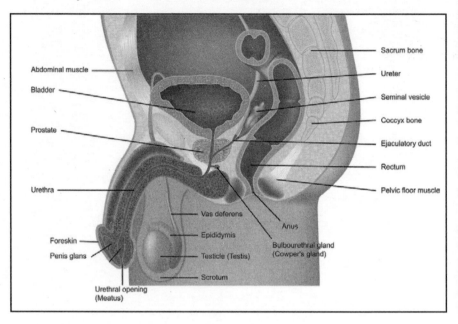

Parts of the male reproductive system

🐾 Penis – This is the male organ used in sexual intercourse. It has three main parts: the root, which connects to the wall of the abdomen; the body; and the glans, which is the cone-shaped part at the end of the penis. The glans, which is also sometimes called the head of the penis, is usually covered with a loose layer of skin called the foreskin. I say usually, because sometimes this skin is removed in a procedure called circumcision. The opening of the urethra, the tube that transports urine and semen, is at the tip of the penis.

The body of the penis is cylindrical and has three circular-shaped chambers. These chambers are made up of sponge-like tissue that contains thousands of gaps that fill with blood when the man becomes sexually aroused. When the penis fills with blood, it becomes rigid and erect, which facilitates penetration during sexual intercourse. When the penis is erect, the flow of urine from the urethra is blocked. This means that only semen, which contains sperm, can be ejaculated during male orgasm. The reason why the skin of the penis is loose is to accommodate changes in penis size during erection.

🖎 Scrotum – This is the pouch or sac-like skin that hangs behind and below the penis. The scrotum contains the testes, or testicles, along with many nerve endings and blood vessels. The scrotum hangs outside the body in order to control the temperature of the testes. To cater for normal sperm development, the testes must be maintained at a temperature slightly cooler than body temperature. Special muscles within the wall of the scrotum enable it to contract or relax, moving the testicles closer to or away from the body for warmth or to cool their temperature.

🖎 Testicles (testes) – These are oval rugby-ball-shaped organs about the size of large olives that lie inside the scrotum. They are connected at either end by a structure called the spermatic cord. Men have two testicles and these are responsible for making testosterone, which is the main male sex hormone, and for generating sperm. Within the testicles are coiled masses of tubes called seminiferous tubules. These tubes are responsible for producing sperm cells.

🖎 Epididymis – This is a long, coiled tube that rests on the backside of each testicle and stores and transports sperm. The sperm that emerge from the testicles are immature and incapable of fertilisation. The epididymis brings these sperm to maturity. During sexual arousal, contractions force the sperm into the vas deferens.

↳ Vas deferens – This is a long, muscular tube that runs from the epididymis into the pelvic cavity, to just behind the bladder. The vas deferens transports the mature sperm to the urethra.

↳ Ejaculatory ducts – These are formed by the merging of the vas deferens and the seminal vesicles. The ejaculatory ducts empty into the urethra.

↳ Urethra – This tube carries urine from the bladder to outside of the body. In males, it has the additional function of ejaculating semen when the man reaches orgasm. When the penis is erect during sex, the flow of urine is blocked so that only semen can be ejaculated at orgasm.

↳ Seminal vesicles – The seminal vesicles are small sac-like pouches that attach to the vas deferens near the base of the bladder. The seminal vesicles produce a sugar-rich fluid (fructose) that provides sperm with a source of energy to help them move. The seminal fluid makes up most of the volume of a man's ejaculate.

↳ Prostate gland – This is a walnut-sized gland that is located below the urinary bladder in front of the rectum. The prostate gland contributes additional fluid to the ejaculate. Fluids from the prostate help to nourish the sperm. The urethra, which then carries the ejaculate to be expelled during orgasm, runs right through the centre of the prostate gland.

↳ Bulbourethral glands – These glands, also known as Cowper's glands, are pea-sized structures located on the sides of the urethra just below the prostate gland. They produce a clear fluid that empties directly into the urethra. This fluid serves to lubricate the urethra and also to neutralise any acidity that may be present due to residual drops of urine in the urethra.

♀♂

How the male reproductive system functions

The functioning of the male reproductive system depends on hormones. The primary hormones involved are follicle-stimulating hormone (FSH), luteinising hormone (LH), and testosterone.

FSH is required for sperm production (spermatogenesis) and LH stimulates the production of testosterone, which is also needed to produce sperm. Testosterone is responsible for the development of male characteristics, including fat distribution, muscle mass, bone mass, facial hair growth, voice change and sex drive. A high FSH level indicates that the body is struggling to produce sperm, as it needs more FSH to perform the task. If the male is easily producing sperm he can do so without FSH levels rising too high. At puberty the testicles produce around 50,000 new sperm every minute of the day and this will continue until a man is in his seventies or even older. Each sperm cell consists of a head, containing the man's genetic code, a mid-section and a tail that helps the sperm swim and penetrate the egg.

Each sperm takes about three months to develop. This means that if a man becomes ill, it can affect his sperm for up to three months. When you implement the Fertility Code it generally takes a few months for sperm quality to improve.

♀ ♂

Male fertility myths

When a couple is experiencing fertility problems, initial thoughts are frequently directed towards the woman. It is often assumed that she can't conceive. However, the man is just as likely to be the issue as the woman. Around 40 per cent of infertility cases are due to low sperm count or quality. Fortunately, the most common causes of male infertility are easy to diagnose, and can be treated.

Myth one – Having sex daily increases your chances of conception

Conception is all about timing. The time you are most likely to conceive is typically from the eleventh to the seventeenth day of a woman's menstrual cycle. Since a man's sperm can live for up to five days in a woman's body, having sex daily will do little to improve fertility. A recent study found practically no difference in pregnancy rates between couples who had sex daily and those who had sex every other day. It is suggested that daily sex may improve the quality of sperm, but that less frequent sex may increase sperm count.

Myth two – Men don't have fertility cycles

Men do have subtle fertility cycles and, generally speaking, the time of year and time of day have an effect on a man's sperm count. Sperm counts are typically higher in winter and lower in summer. This is probably because sperm production increases in cooler temperatures. Sperm counts are also usually highest in the morning when male hormone levels are at their peak.

Myth three – All exercise is good for male fertility

We will look at exercise in more detail later in this book but, generally speaking, too much exercise is harmful for both male and female fertility. Cycling in particular has come under some scrutiny. Sitting on a bicycle saddle for more than thirty minutes at a time, especially if wearing tight bicycle shorts, can raise scrotal temperature, which temporarily affects sperm production because the scrotum is pushed closer to the body. For the same reason it is also recommended that men hoping to conceive should avoid taking hot baths, or using hot tubs and saunas.

Myth four – Lubricants can help conception

Although lubricants decrease friction and can increase the pleasure of sex, they will not help you get pregnant. In fact, some lubricants can be unhelpful because they can interfere with sperm motility and some contain ingredients that are harmful to sperm. If you need to use a lubricant for sex, make sure to consult your doctor or pharmacist and use an intimate moisturiser that does not interfere with your chances of conception.

Myth five – When it comes to weight, only being overweight affects sperm

Male obesity can affect sperm production, but being too thin can also reduce sperm count. Being underweight is understood to affect sperm because the condition is linked to hormonal imbalances as well as malnutrition. The 2008 European Society of Human Reproduction and Embryology conference in Barcelona presented studies that showed that men of optimal weight had higher levels of normal sperm than those who were either overweight or underweight. The Fertility Code Nutrition Plan should assist you in achieving your optimal weight if you are not at the right weight already.

Male fertility investigation

Evaluation of male fertility should begin with a visit to a urologist. The urologist will likely start with a physical examination and an interview covering the following information:

- ♫ A full medical and reproductive history, along with evaluation of any surgeries or medications taken
- ♫ Questions about lifestyle, including exercise, smoking, and drug use
- ♫ A frank discussion about your sexual life, including any problems with sex or previous sexually transmitted diseases

The man will need to provide a semen sample for analysis. The doctor will usually want the man to give the sample there on site, as it is helpful for the analysis to take place quickly.

Male fertility tests

Sperm and semen analysis

A urologist assesses the man's sperm count, their shape, movement, and other variables. The higher the number of normal-shaped sperm, the more fertile the man generally is. There are, however, exceptions and many men with low sperm counts or abnormal semen can still be quite fertile and not encounter any problems conceiving. Also, it is estimated that about 15 per cent of men with fertility problems have normal semen and plenty of normal sperm.

If the first semen analysis is normal, the doctor may perform a second test to confirm the results. Two normal tests are generally interpreted as indicating that the man does not have any significant fertility problems. If something in the results looks irregular, the doctor will usually also order further tests to confirm the precise problem.

If no semen or sperm are present (azoospermia), this may not be so bad, as corrective surgery could remove a blockage in the 'plumbing' and rectify the problem.

A sperm-count test looks at the total number of sperm and also how those sperm swim, the direction in which they swim, and their shape and size. The sperm-count analysis also looks at the semen colour, how it clumps together, how much semen volume there is and many other factors.

A sperm culture may be done, which can identify any signs of infection.

According to the World Health Organization, a sperm concentration of twenty million per millilitre, and a total of at least forty million per ejaculate, is needed for optimum fertility. In some cases, however, the number of sperm may be normal, but other factors are preventing pregnancy occurring.

If the results obtained are abnormal, the next step is typically to find out where things are going wrong, and if possible, correct the problem or problems. If the problem cannot be fixed, fertility treatments may be suggested.

Sometimes sperm test results can be difficult to understand. A sperm count result may fall above normal on one scale and below normal on another. As always, speak to your doctor if you don't understand the results of your test.

Sperm health depends on several factors, including:

- ↳ Sperm count (quantity) – You are most likely to be fertile if the semen discharged in a single ejaculation contains more than thirty-nine million sperm.

✤ Sperm morphology (quality) – You are most likely to be fertile if more than 4 per cent of your sperm have a normal structure and shape. A normal sperm has an oval head and a long tail, which work together to propel it forward. Sperm with large, small, tapered or crooked heads with curled or double tails are less likely to fertilise an egg.

✤ Sperm vitality (motility) – In order for the sperm to reach the egg they must move on their own, swimming the last few inches to reach and penetrate the egg. You are most likely to be fertile if more than 40 per cent of your sperm are moving.

Physical examination

A good physical exam will detect abnormal veins or varicoceles above the testicles. Varicoceles are the most common cause of correctable male infertility accounting for up to 38 per cent of cases. These abnormal formations of veins above the testicle can be fixed with surgery.

Other potential sperm issues

Abnormal anti-sperm antibodies (ASA)

Some men make abnormal anti-sperm antibodies (ASA) against their own sperm. These antibodies attack the sperm on the way to the egg and can prevent fertilisation. Anti-sperm antibodies happen when the body becomes sensitive to sperm, causing an immune system response that destroys the sperm. Normally sperm is protected from the immune system by way of a barrier in the testes. However, with men who have anti-sperm antibodies, this barrier has somehow been broken, allowing the immune cells to have access to and damage the sperm.

Sperm can be affected in a variety of ways, depending on where the antibodies are located. When the antibodies are found on the tail, sperm can be immobilised or can clump together. Antibodies positioned on the head can prevent the sperm from binding properly to the egg, which prevents fertilisation taking place.

A woman's cervical mucus can also sometimes develop antibodies to her partner's sperm. It is believed that anti-sperm antibodies in the cervical mucus may account for as much as 40 per cent of unexplained infertility in couples.

Causes of anti-sperm antibodies

There are a number of possible reasons why anti-sperm antibodies occur. Anything that causes a disruption to the natural barrier between sperm and the immune system can increase the likelihood of ASAs. Some common causes include:

- ♮ Infection
- ♮ Undescended testicles
- ♮ Twisting or injury to the testicles
- ♮ Testicular cancer
- ♮ Varicocele

Men who have had a vasectomy reversal are especially likely to have anti-sperm antibodies. Almost 70 per cent of men who undergo this procedure have anti-sperm antibodies.

Treatment

When production of anti-sperm antibodies has been identified as a fertility issue affecting either the man or the woman, there are a number of excellent assisted reproductive treatment approaches that can address this issue. These might include intrauterine insemination (IUI), intracytoplasmic sperm injection (ICSI) or in vitro fertilisation (IVF) treatment.

In addition there are things you can do for yourself which may alter the production of these ASAs.

Channels of elimination

Your body relies on all possible channels of elimination when it comes to getting rid of toxins. They are mostly mucus- and discharge-producing organs such as the nose, lungs, skin, kidneys, gut, vagina and penis. The fluids discharged are known in Chinese medicine as jin ye – precious liquid – a term used to describe all the liquids in the body. Jin ye protects, nourishes and lubricates. The jin are the lighter-weight fluids that moisten and nourish the skin and muscles, while the ye are the thicker, more viscous fluids of the bones, organs, brain and body orifices. Sweat, tears, saliva, urine, joint lubricant, spinal fluid, semen and breast milk are some of the bodily fluids that make up jin ye.

Your body is on average 60 per cent fluid. It is also dependent on fluid to flush toxins out of vital organs, carry nutrients to your cells, and provide a moist environment for ear, nose and throat tissues.

When the body's fluid metabolism is disrupted, jin ye can accumulate and thicken into phlegm.

Too much fire dries you up.
Too much water drains you out.
This imbalance can be controlled
only by cultivating equilibrium.

Chang Po-Tuan, Taoist master (A.D. 983–1082)

This is where the Fertility Code Detox, discussed later in this book, comes into the picture. Every couple, whether encountering fertility issues or not, should clean their nutrition and consider detoxing before conception. This is how you improve the quality of these fluids and cultivate equilibrium, or balance.

Exposure to heavy metals and other toxins have a detrimental impact on the immune system, especially on autoantibody production, which can lead to infertility in susceptible individuals. One study found that patients with mercury allergy had more anti-sperm antibodies than patients without mercury allergy. (Neuro. Endicronol. Lett., 2005)

♀♂

Food intolerances and anti-sperm antibodies

If the immune system is in overdrive (due to constant exposure to foods you are intolerant to) it can adversely react to sperm. This can lead to creation of antibodies to sperm in both men and women and can predispose the woman to miscarriage.

You will not necessarily know that you have a food intolerance until you do a proper blood test or, if you have symptoms, you simply eliminate the food from your diet and wait to see if the symptoms go away. Chinese medicine's understanding is that if you produce a lot of phlegm or experience sinus or digestive problems, these can be indications that you have compromised your fluid system, perhaps through your diet.

After a couple implements the Fertility Code Nutrition and Detox Plans, it can take up to three months for the immune-complexes (antibodies and antigens sticking together) to clear from your system.

Reducing anti-sperm antibodies in women

If a woman's mucus is confirmed to contain anti-sperm antibodies and this is believed to be the main issue causing the fertility problem, more than just good nutrition and a detox are suggested. Studies have shown that women can develop anti-sperm antibodies if sperm has come into contact with the systemic immune system. This can happen if there are minor cuts or wounds in the vagina or the oral cavity. Sperm antibodies in cervical mucus cause the heads of the sperm to stick to the cervical mucus.

You can treat female sperm antibodies by using condoms and avoiding oral sex for three to six months. This allows the woman's immune system to improve with diet and nutritional supplements. Because the woman doesn't come into contact with any sperm during this time, the antibodies to sperm will break down and no new ones will be produced. This is also a good time to try to determine when your most fertile days are.

After this period, you stop using condoms and have intercourse at your most fertile time. This does not allow enough time for the woman to produce new antibodies and because the woman's immune system has been improved and retrained during those three to six months, it is likely that it will not react the same way when it encounters sperm.

If sperm antibodies are found in the woman's blood, then just relying on using condoms will not be enough and a longer immune system treatment may be suggested.

Reducing anti-sperm antibodies in men

Autoimmunity is the result of an abnormal immune response against the body's own tissue. When men develop antibodies against their own sperm it can cause the sperm to stick together (agglutinate), or cause the tails of the sperm to stick to the cervical mucus. This issue with autoimmunity may have existed from birth or even before or as a result of digestive problems frequently associated with improper diet.

Autoimmunity of any form can derive from early childhood or from development in the womb. If the mother was consuming foods to which she was intolerant during her pregnancy, then her antibodies influenced what type of immune system dominance the child would have. Chinese medicine has understood this for thousands of years and says that the best time to treat someone is the *year before* they are born. In other words if both parents are healthy prior to conception, this will help to deliver good health for their offspring that will last throughout their life.

If a child was not breastfed, this can hamper the development of a healthy immune system, as some of the mother's antibodies may not have been passed on, which can predispose the child to an immune system that is overly reactive.

A faulty immune system can also occur as a result of improper diet and can lead to inflammation in the gut. This can be as a result of food intolerances or due to a bacterial or parasitic infection. Symptoms of this include bloating, excessive wind, bowel irregularities and fatigue. In this case large molecules from food may have entered the sterile environment behind the gut, through the gaps between the cell walls. This is commonly known as leaky gut. Once these food molecules are in the area of the body they are not meant to be in, the immune system will pick them up and treat them as invading pathogens. Now that the immune system has been exposed to this substance once, it may well produce a whole army of antibodies against this food. So each time you eat this food, the antibodies enter attack mode. In this attack mode the immune system can attack other cells it sees as threatening, including sperm cells. Over time this will exhaust the immune reserve, making it weaker when it comes to dealing with bacteria and viruses. The person will then frequently become hypersensitive to his or her own tissue and innocuous substances such as pollen and food.

♀ ♂

Three steps to help correct a faulty immune system

↳ Detoxify the identifiable triggers for three to six months or longer, depending on the severity; typical triggers are dairy, wheat etc.

↳ Heal the inflammation and the mucosal surfaces with the Fertility Code Nutrition Plan.

↳ Treat the immune system with adequate protein intake, ongoing clean diet, and support with the Fertility Code supplements.

Other structural challenges

In some men, making sperm isn't the problem – it's getting the sperm to where they need to go that poses the difficulty. Some men have normal sperm in their testicles. The sperm in the semen, though, are missing, very low in number, or abnormal. There are several reasons for low sperm in semen when a man is making enough sperm.

↳ Retrograde ejaculation is a condition where sperm ejaculates backwards, into the bladder. Usually retrograde ejaculation is caused by a previous surgery.

↳ Absence of the main sperm pipeline (the vas

deferens) – a genetic problem that some men are born with.

🖎 Obstruction anywhere between the testicles and the penis.

🖎 Anti-sperm antibodies attacking a man's own sperm on their way to the egg.

♀♂

Creating healthy sperm

The following simple steps have been identified as critical to improving sperm health. If there is no structural impediment to conceiving (and even if there is), it makes complete sense to implement these measures.

What you should do

🖎 Eat plenty of fruits and vegetables. These foods are rich in antioxidants, which help to improve sperm health.

🖎 Manage stress. Stress interferes with certain hormones needed to produce sperm. Stress can also decrease sexual desire and function.

🖎 Get the appropriate amount of exercise. Physical activity is good for reproductive health as well as overall health, but don't overdo it. If you exercise to exhaustion, you may experience a temporary change in hormone levels and a drop in sperm quality.

🖎 Watch your weight. Too much body fat may disrupt production of reproductive hormones, which can reduce your sperm count and increase your percentage of abnormal sperm. You are much more likely to produce high-quality sperm if you maintain a healthy weight.

✤ Take supplements. Taking Fertility Code
multivitamins and supplements daily will ensure that
you are getting the nutrients that are important for
optimal sperm production and function.

What you should avoid

Sperm can also be vulnerable to environmental factors, such
as exposure to excessive heat or toxic chemicals. To protect your
fertility you should take the following measures.

✤ Avoid tobacco. If you smoke, do what you need to
do to quit. Smoking causes sperm to be misshapen
and slow. In addition, smoking can damage your
sperm's DNA, possibly affecting a baby's growth and
development, and increasing the risk of cancer.

✤ Limit alcohol. Heavy drinking can reduce the quality
and quantity of sperm. If you choose to drink alcohol,
limit yourself to no more than one or two drinks a day.

✤ Steer clear of recreational drugs. Marijuana decreases
sperm motility and increases the number of abnormal
sperm. Cocaine and opiates can contribute to erectile
dysfunction and a host of sexual problems.

✤ Skip the bath. Spending more than thirty minutes in
hot water that is 40°C or above is likely to lower your
sperm count. Avoid hot tubs, steamy baths and saunas
for the same reason.

✤ Limit your time on the bike. Cycling for more than
thirty minutes at a time – especially if you also
wear tight bicycle shorts – may raise your scrotal
temperature and affect sperm production. If you
cycle, choose a saddle that's not too hard or narrow,
and make sure it's adjusted to keep your weight on
your 'sit bones'. While you're biking, stop for frequent
rests.

- ✤ Avoid lubricants during sex. Personal lubricants, lotions and even saliva can interfere with sperm motility. If it is necessary to use a lubricant seek the advice of your doctor or pharmacist and look for an intimate moisturiser that won't harm sperm.

- ✤ Get medical advice on medications. Steroids, antibiotics and certain medications used to control chronic conditions, such as high blood pressure or inflammatory bowel disease, can reduce your fertility. Anti-androgens used to treat prostate enlargement and cancer interfere with sperm production. These medications may be necessary, so seek the advice of your doctor, indicating your wish to optimise fertility, before making any adjustments. In addition, chemotherapy drugs and radiation treatment for cancer can cause permanent infertility. If you're considering cancer treatment, consider saving and freezing your sperm (semen cryopreservation) beforehand.

- ✤ Watch out for toxins. Workplace and household substances such as industrial heavy metals, pesticides and chemicals in solvents may affect sperm quantity and quality. Avoid these where possible and when they cannot be avoided use protective clothing, good ventilation and facemasks to reduce the risk of absorbing toxins.

Case study – Jennifer and Michael

Jennifer and Michael had been trying to conceive for three years without success. After they had undergone a series of tests it was established that there was no impediment to conception with regard to Jennifer, but that Michael had sperm quality and quantity issues. Both attended the clinic and together they decided to implement lifestyle changes to optimise their fertility. Michael had quite a stressful job, which for him meant that he frequently ate on the run and usually not the best food. As a consequence he needed to pay particular attention to his weight.

Although he was overweight, he was also malnourished in the sense that his diet wasn't providing him with the nutrients necessary for optimal health and fertility. This is a very common scenario.

Michael was determined to make changes that would improve his health. After a few weeks he began to notice that he had more energy. He used this energy to exercise more and he started sleeping better. Within two short months he had lost almost 20 lbs, which in turn made him feel better. A vicious circle had very quickly become a virtuous circle. Three months after they started the programme Michael repeated the sperm analysis, which now showed a marked improvement in the results. This gave him the encouragement to continue with the programme and two months later Jennifer successfully conceived. Four years on Jennifer and Michael are the proud parents of two boys.

WHEN TO HAVE SEX – TIMING AND FREQUENCY

The most important factor affecting your chances of conceiving is something that you and your partner have complete control over: the timing and frequency of intercourse during your fertile window.

What is the fertile window?

The fertile window is the period of days during the menstrual cycle when pregnancy is possible. The length of this fertile phase is primarily determined by the maximum life span of the sperm. Sperm can survive a maximum of five days within a woman's fertile cervical fluid and the woman's egg, or ovum, can survive for up to one day. In theory therefore the fertile window is a maximum of six days long: the five days before ovulation and the day of ovulation. You can only conceive naturally when you have intercourse on one of these days. Although pregnancy is possible from intercourse on any one of these six days, the likelihood of actually becoming pregnant is dramatically increased when you have intercourse in the three days immediately leading up to and including ovulation. This means that in practical terms the fertile window is more like three days.

Predicting ovulation

There are a few ways to time intercourse. One simple approach is to have intercourse every second day between days eight and eighteen of the woman's cycle, counting day one as the first day of the period. This will almost certainly cover the fertile window, when ovulation should occur.

You can also detect ovulation by keeping track of changes in cervical mucus, the fluid normally released from the vagina. At the beginning of the menstrual cycle, this mucus should be relatively sparse, dense and tacky, but around the fertile window it becomes increasingly plentiful and slippery, similar to the white of a raw egg.

Many of my fellow acupuncturists are particularly fond of tracking ovulation by charting and using body temperature as an indicator. This is known as the Basal Body Temperature Method. It identifies ovulation from changes in body temperature (a rise of .5°C to 1.6°C after a woman ovulates). This method I particularly dislike. First of all it doesn't predict ovulation at all, only indicating ovulation after it has already occurred, which might be too late. More significantly, it encourages an unhealthy, obsessive focus on fertility that often creates a whole new level of stress and anxiety. Stress and anxiety hamper fertility and therefore I would actively discourage couples from using this method.

Home ovulation prediction kits are more effective and far less stressful. An ovulation predictor kit will give you advance notice of about a day to a day and a half. They work by detecting the pre-ovulation LH surge in your body and predict, with great accuracy, your most fertile time of the month.

When selecting a test, I recommend opting for one that is easy to use and reasonably priced. Most of the tests are used in the same way – all you do is hold the stick tester in your urine stream for several seconds, then wait five minutes for the results.

For the first few months I still think it is better to simply have sex before the time you think you will be ovulating and let the whole process be as relaxed as possible. If after a few months of actively trying, you want to predict ovulation, then I would suggest using an ovulation predictor test.

A 1995 study by the National Institute of Environmental Health Sciences confirmed that a woman's fertile window lasts six days: the five days leading up to, and the day of, ovulation. What's more, the study showed that the likelihood of pregnancy decreased from about 36 per cent (if intercourse occurred two days before and/or on the day of ovulation) to 10 per cent (if it occurred four to six days before). Since sperm can survive for up to five days, 'old' sperm can fertilise an egg, but it is far less likely.

How often should you have sex?

There are differing opinions when it comes to this question. One school of thought is that you should have intercourse as frequently as possible to increase your chances of conception. The logic is fairly straightforward: the more you have sex, the more likely it is that the timing will coincide with the optimum time within the fertile window.

Another long-held view was that a man should abstain from sex for several days prior to the fertile window in order to build up his sperm count. Part of this presumption is true and studies have shown that the more frequently a man ejaculates over a period of several days, the lower his sperm count.

But this, as it turns out, appears not to matter. Although a man's sperm count may decrease the more often he has intercourse, it should still be high enough to achieve pregnancy. The Environmental Health Sciences study found that the more sex you have, the greater your chances of getting pregnant (Wilcox et al, 2000). Dr. Wilcox, the senior researcher in the study, found that couples who had intercourse every other day during their fertile days still had very high odds of conceiving, specifically, a 22 per cent chance of conception per cycle. This compares well with 25 per cent for those who had sex every day. However, couples who had sex once per week reduced their chances of conception to 10 per cent, since they were more likely to miss the key baby-making window of opportunity.

Therefore, frequent intercourse within a narrow fertile window increases your chances of conception and can ultimately reduce the time it takes to conceive.

Am I pregnant?

For most couples, the first clue to pregnancy comes in a pretty obvious form: a missed period. But some women claim that, even before skipping a period, they feel pregnant – that is, they experience a range of symptoms, including fatigue, headaches, queasiness, bloating, breast tenderness, mild cramps, some skin issues, heightened sensitivity to smells and an increased urge to urinate.

Of course, the best way to confirm pregnancy is to use a home pregnancy test, making sure to wait at least until your period was due. Testing any earlier than this can result in a false negative, even if pregnancy has occurred. If the home test indicates pregnancy, most people will want to check with their doctor, who will generally perform a further test after you have missed a period. This will confirm pregnancy with absolute certainty.

Of course, if you are pregnant you should continue to implement the Fertility Code. The goal is to have a healthy and happy baby and implementing the Fertility Code will help you towards that goal.

If you are not pregnant

If you are relatively young – in your late twenties to early thirties – you don't necessarily have to rush to a fertility specialist if you're finding it difficult to conceive. You should, however, make sure that you are taking the correct approach to optimising your chances of fertility. There are two common mistakes that couples make.

> ✍ Wasting too much time before consulting a fertility specialist – Many couples keep the dreaded basal body temperature charts for six months before they consult their doctor or order any tests. Your doctor or gynaecologist should take a detailed health history from both the man and the woman, which may

reveal clues as to why you are having difficulties.
He or she is likely to perform a semen analysis and
provide instruction in using ovulation kits. A fertility
specialist will also help to identify if there are medical
reasons that might be causing you difficulties in
achieving pregnancy. Conditions that can present
obstacles to fertility, such as endometriosis, PCOS
and a myriad of others, can be identified and then a
sensible and informed approach can follow.

- Mistiming tests – A blood test of the level of serum
  progesterone (the hormone that readies your uterus
  for implantation of the fertilised egg) should be taken
  exactly seven days after ovulation. A post-coital
  exam (a check of the quality of your cervical mucus
  and how well sperm penetrates it) has to occur after
  intercourse and within twenty-four hours of when
  your LH level surges. Too often these tests are based
  on a hypothetical twenty-eight-day cycle, rather than
  the results of home ovulation monitoring.

♀♂

CHAPTER SUMMARY

- When you've decided that you want to start a family
  it often seems like everyone around you is expecting.
  The truth, however, is that getting pregnant often isn't
  as simple as you imagined and it is estimated that one
  in three people encounter stress and anxiety related
  to fertility. Give yourself time!

- If you are under thirty-five and actively trying to
  conceive, I would suggest that you seek medical
  advice after twelve months of unprotected sex. If you
  are over thirty-five I would suggest you seek advice
  after four to six months.

- ♮ Age isn't the only factor; equally important is good health. This is why the Fertility Code can significantly increase your chances.

- ♮ Knowing when ovulation occurs is important if you want to increase the likelihood of conception. There are a number of ways to predict the timing of ovulation, but in my opinion, by far the best and least stressful way is to use ovulation predictor kits.

- ♮ When a couple is encountering fertility problems, a male factor is just as likely to be the issue as a female factor. Frequently these male factor issues can be treated and they often respond well to lifestyle changes.

- ♮ Have sex frequently during your fertile window, but it doesn't need to be too often. There is only a marginal advantage to having sex every day during this time, compared to every other day. Having sex more than once a day could even be detrimental, as it may lower sperm count.

- ♮ If you get pregnant soon after commencing the Fertility Code continue with the programme, as this is also an optimal approach for a successful pregnancy and a healthy baby.

THE
Fertility CODE
Mind Programme

"The energy of the mind is the essence of life"

Aristotle

INTRODUCTION

If you are reading this book there is a strong chance that fertility has caused stress or anxiety in your life. You may feel very alone with these emotions despite the fact that one in six couples experiences similar challenges. For some people the mental and emotional impact of trying to conceive can take hold very quickly, within the first few months. You may have been given a medical diagnosis stating that there are real physical barriers to having a baby. However, becoming stressed about your fertility creates a further impediment to your goal. Whatever your position, you wish to enhance your chances of a successful pregnancy and a healthy baby, and developing the correct mental framework has to be central to achieving this. The Fertility Code Mind Programme will help to deliver optimal psychology for conception.

I have worked with thousands of patients over the years, dealing with a variety of conditions, some of them life threatening. However, I have found that the psychological impact of fertility problems can be so profound that it frequently affects a person's physical and emotional well-being far more than other potentially more serious conditions. It is quite easy for a vicious circle to develop, where fertility problems lead to stress and then the stress exacerbates those fertility issues. One Harvard study led by Dr Alice Domar showed that women who had addressed stress issues by completing a mind-body programme or participating in a support group were almost three times as likely to get pregnant within a year, compared with those who received medical treatment alone (Domar et al, 2000). Another study showed that women who participated in a stress management programme before or during their IVF cycle had a 160 per cent greater success rate than those who did not (Domar et al, 2011). A 2009 study by the European Society of Reproduction and Embryology showed that stressful life events experienced within twelve months of IVF treatment are a significant predictor of success in achieving pregnancy.

This chapter will provide you with the skills to deal with the emotional aspect of fertility. By performing the exercises contained in this chapter you will empower yourself to reduce the impact of stress and emotional factors related to fertility or affecting your fertility. By working through this programme you will learn to be more at ease with yourself and in control of your emotions. Importantly, by doing this you should also significantly increase your chances of a successful pregnancy.

Although you can work through the exercises in sequence as they are presented here, my suggestion is that you treat this as an ongoing programme and repeat them frequently to improve the way you deal with stress in your daily life. In doing this you will train yourself to become instinctively more at ease. The more you practise these exercises the more in control you will be, and these skills will not only be helpful now, when you are trying to have a baby, but also in the future, whatever life brings you.

♀♂

THE MIND-BODY CONNECTION

If you have been trying to have a baby for some time it is more than likely that you have heard the annoying comment, *Just relax and it will happen*. As irritating as this might be, there is some truth in it. But as with comments like, *Don't look so sad*, or, *Cheer up; it might never happen*, the suggestion is that you should feel or act differently, as if it were a simple decision.

The truth is that your mind is central to the functioning of your body. Your brain performs two major types of function: those you are consciously aware of and those we refer to as functions of the subconscious. Essentially the mind is like an iceberg. The visible part of the iceberg is like our conscious mind, but the subconscious mind is far more extensive and is responsible for the key functions central to your continued existence. Your subconscious mind is responsible twenty-four hours a day, seven days a week for maintaining your heartbeat, breathing, digestion, repairing damage to your body, growing your hair and nails, controlling your muscles to coordinate every single movement, as well as regulating your body's temperature, water content and sugar levels. In addition to all of this, it controls your body's regeneration, including growing a complete new skeleton each year, brand-new soft tissue every three months, a new liver every six weeks, eight square metres of new skin every four weeks and a new stomach lining every five days. In fact, 98 per cent of cells in your body are replaced every year.

So it is inevitable that your mind has a profound impact on your health and your fertility. If we accept this, then we should accept that factors such as stress, anxiety and depression not only have an impact on your mental health, but also on your physical health and your fertility.

For many years Western medical practice has separated the mind and body and understated the impact of thought and emotion on physical processes. This began when René Descartes declared, Cogito, ergo sum – I think, therefore I am. Descartes' position was that the mind was distinct from the brain, which in turn was distinct from the body. This philosophy supported a belief in the existence of a soul and therefore was consistent with religious doctrine at the time. Being inconsistent with religious doctrine in seventeenth century France was a dangerous thing. The Catholic Church held the belief that the body was the temple of the soul and therefore any human dissections, and sometimes even operations, were fundamentally at odds with religious doctrine. Separating mind and body philosophically facilitated medical practitioners. Even though Descartes remained a Catholic all his life and firmly believed in the immortal soul, his works were still declared damnable by the Church in 1663.

It seems strange that Descartes' thoughts on the separation of mind and body have dominated medical beliefs until recent times, long after such threats of religious interference in medical advancement have subsided. This philosophy has begun to give way as we increasingly come to understand the intimate connection between mind and body. Traditional Chinese medicine has always held the belief that mind and body are just two sides of the same coin and are completely interconnected. Nowadays medical practitioners and fertility clinics will often recommend or even offer counselling or stress-reduction services to their patients as an integral part of fertility treatment.

♀ ♂

Fight or flight

The relationship between stress and fertility is complicated but it is safe to say that stress, when not properly dealt with, has a negative impact on your fertility. You are probably familiar with the fight-or-flight reaction. This phrase, coined by Walter Bradford Cannon in 1932, describes the natural phenomenon where, faced with danger, the body directs its resources towards one thing – survival. In doing so, heart rate increases, breathing accelerates and becomes shallow, adrenaline and cortisol are released to help us to react quicker and even be stronger. Crucially, other functions unnecessary for our survival are placed on hold. Digestion shuts down, blood vessels constrict and levels of reproductive hormones drop. As we have already discussed, in order to conceive and carry a baby, your hormones must function properly. The correct balance of hormones is required for both males and females to function properly in relation to fertility.

Obviously, you're not trying to have a baby in a fight-or-flight situation, but it is still relevant. Our bodies and subconscious mind can be quite poor at determining what is dangerous and what is not. The stresses associated with modern-day living and the cut and thrust of high-pressure careers are often interpreted by our subconscious as mortal dangers and the fight-or-flight response is activated unnecessarily. In the past we may have needed that response to escape a sabre tooth tiger, but our modern-day stresses are more constant and pervasive. Because of this we are prone to activating this emergency mode in our everyday lives, and if we don't manage this stress response it takes a profound toll.

The physical reactions to stress come from the way it activates the hypothalamus and the adrenal glands. The hypothalamus coordinates the functions of the nervous and hormonal systems for the entire body. It is connected to the pituitary gland through a short connection of nerve fibres and controls the secretions from this gland. During stress the adrenal glands will over-produce adrenaline and cortisol. Familiar symptoms are digestive problems, tense muscles (particularly in the shoulders) and raised blood pressure. The excessive production of adrenaline and cortisol interferes with the production of hormones, including follicle stimulating hormone (FSH) and luteinising hormone (LH), in both men and women. The decreases in FSH and LH results in a lowering of testosterone, oestrogen and progesterone, all of which play a critical role in conception and successful implantation. Prolactin is another hormone released by the pituitary gland in situations of physical or emotional stress, and high levels of this hormone can stop a woman's menstrual cycle and cause impotence in men. Such imbalances can also cause the fallopian tubes and the uterus to contract, inhibiting the movement of the egg to the uterus.

In men, emotional stress is associated with abnormal sperm development. A recent Turkish study revealed that medical students prior to their final exams had lower sperm counts, lower motility and a higher percentage of sperm abnormality compared with the same students when they were not under the same stress. The study also revealed that fertility was restored soon after the exams were over and the stress had disappeared.

Additional research from the University of California, Berkeley adds backing to the benefits to male fertility when stress is managed. When stress hormones like cortisol are increased it triggers a decrease in the production of gonadotropin releasing hormone (GnRH). This in turn affects the production of other key hormones, LH and FSH, which can directly affect the quantity and quality of sperm.

The emotional roller coaster

The instinct to mate and to then protect one's offspring can go beyond the survival instinct. Therefore it shouldn't be a surprise that couples encountering fertility problems often experience extreme stress if they believe they may not be able to produce a family.

Menstruation can bring with it a host of feelings. Before trying for a baby, the feeling may have been predominantly relief, the assumption being that pregnancy was something that could easily happen if you were not careful. But now that pregnancy is yearned for, the feeling of relief may be replaced with emotions of sadness, grief, frustration, anger and inadequacy. These feelings can shake the very core of your being and it is natural that you will want to share what you are feeling with someone, and, typically, that will be your partner. However, whilst a man can feel sympathy because his partner is upset, I don't believe he can truly appreciate the depth of these feelings. This in itself can put a strain on the relationship. For a woman it can sometimes appear that her partner is simply not overly concerned and comments like, Don't worry; it could happen next month, can easily be misinterpreted as, I'm not worried.

The truth is that men are not programmed to feel the same as women do about childbearing. Of course most men do want to reproduce, but they do not grow up with an expectation that they will get pregnant. Pregnancy is something they will never experience and so they do not have the same emotional involvement in the ability to get pregnant that a woman naturally has. From the time she was a little girl, frequently playing with dolls, a woman has been encouraged to act out the role of a mother.

Male psychology and fertility

If the fertility problem is down to a male factor, a whole other dynamic is introduced. For the male psyche the ability to reproduce is often intertwined with belief in his sexual prowess. The emotional charge attached to this situation can be intense. Fertility problems can make men feel weak and inadequate. Whilst a woman experiencing fertility challenges will want to share her feelings, a man, already feeling a sense of weakness, may perceive sharing his feelings as a further sign of frailty. For this reason, at my clinic it is the norm for the woman to seek assistance even though it has already been determined that the man's fertility is the problem factor and it is he who would benefit more from treatment.

In this situation we have a woman with a deep yearning to have baby and a desire to share her feelings and we have a man with equally deep feelings of frailty. We also have on his part a determination to keep as stoic as possible lest he increase his vulnerability further. Many men fear that talking about the difficulty will make their position even worse and they may seek to avoid the subject completely or withdraw when it is brought up. They might even have an unspoken fear that this problem will cost them their relationship, something that perhaps terrifies them. Again, this silence is often misinterpreted as a lack of concern and it is likely to make the woman feel resentment. If you are a woman in this position you can be pretty certain that your partner is going through deep inner turmoil well beyond your perception. Awareness of this fact can be helpful for a lot of women. The fact that he doesn't want to discuss it, or doesn't know how to comfort his partner, does not mean that a man's emotions are any less painful.

Emotional strain can also occur when you seek the comfort of friends and family and it doesn't seem to be there. The strain is compounded by friends and work colleagues all around you getting pregnant and having babies. For many women the challenge that this presents can often seem overwhelming and it is not helped by the natural tendency of mothers to talk incessantly about their babies and children. Your family members may also be so busy having babies and coping with bringing up their children that they appear not to empathise with you. This can lead to feelings of resentment and sometimes loneliness.

As the months pass and you are still waiting to become pregnant, there are further opportunities to hear about other women's pregnancies. This can become almost intolerable and you may find yourself avoiding social gatherings and events that will put you in contact with women who are expecting or already have children. It is not uncommon for women to completely withdraw from almost all social activity because of this difficulty. Of course when this happens, feelings of loneliness only increase.

♀♂

UNDERSTANDING WORRY

The word 'worry' is derived from the Old English word 'wyrgan' which means 'to strangle' or 'to choke'. This is in essence what worry does to us. It strangles the life out of us. Medical research has shown that worry breaks down our resistance to disease and can cause a multiplicity of health issues. Apart from physical ill-health, it affects our overall enjoyment of life, putting us in a bad mood, hurting our relationships and robbing us of zest, energy and optimism.

However, exploring the actual content of your worries, as well as the psychological tendencies that might be contributing to this worry, will allow you to gain greater understanding and control of your emotions. In Chinese medicine, worry is perceived as overthinking. This is a condition in which you are preoccupied with thinking about your feelings rather than feeling your feelings. These thoughts frequently go round and round in circles, depleting your mental and physical energy.

Common worries

It is often helpful to understand that you are not alone with your worry. The worries you have are likely to be shared with many people in a similar position. Other people have had these same worries and have come through them successfully. Another aspect worth considering is the reality that many worries are pointless. It has been estimated that:

- 40 per cent of things we worry about will never actually happen

- 30 per cent are things in the past we cannot change

- 12 per cent relate to other people's concerns that we cannot influence

- 10 per cent relate to our health even when in fact nothing is wrong.

This means that just 8 per cent of the things we worry about are genuinely concerning. Even in these situations, expending energy on worry usually does nothing to alter the situation.

Yale University researchers have actually discovered a 'worry gene'. However although this gene can be passed on by your parents, that doesn't mean that you can't overcome it.

Self-dialogue and worry

I have frequently heard clients describe themselves as worriers, as if this was part and parcel of who they were as people and it was an aspect of themselves they could not change. I don't accept that this has to be the case. Worrying may be almost a way of life for some people, however, it has its roots in a self-dialogue that can be changed.

How does worry affect fertility?

Recent studies have found that women who experience worry and anxiety have reduced blood flow to their uterus and ovaries. If this is severe it can cause a decrease in the number of viable eggs produced by the ovaries and have an impact on the quality of the uterine lining. Doctors from the Queen Charlotte's and Chelsea Hospital in London studied one hundred expectant mothers and found that pregnant women who were more anxious had significantly abnormal patterns of blood flow through the uterine arteries. The findings, published in the British Medical Journal, suggested that 'the psychological state of the mother may affect foetal development and therefore birth weight'.

Dr Vivette Glover, one of the authors of the study, believes that this research indicates that even small variations in birth weight caused by anxiety could have a potentially serious impact on health in later life. We do not fully understand why worry can affect fertility and pregnancy, but one suggestion is that worry raises the levels of hormones such as noradrenaline, which is known to constrict the blood vessels and decrease blood flow. Another possibility is that anxiety may have a chemical effect on the development of the blood vessels early in pregnancy.

Changing the voices in your head

From the time we wake in the morning we begin a constant self-dialogue. Indeed it is safe to say that this conversation continues at a subconscious level even while we sleep. Many of us are in the habit of being very harsh on ourselves; whenever we make even a minor blunder we admonish ourselves in the most ruthless manner imaginable. Most people would not tolerate being spoken to by anyone else in the manner in which they speak to themselves. The problem with this ruthless self-dialogue is that it has a significant impact on the way we feel mentally, emotionally and even physically. In order to understand how we are thinking, we need to look at this self-dialogue. By becoming aware of the words and phrases you use, your tone of voice and the intention behind your words, you will learn to understand the programming code of your own brain. It is these words that are actually controlling your mind, and it is only by altering these words that you can effectively change the way you think – and change the way you handle stress and anxiety.

Take some time now to consider the manner in which you talk to yourself. Negative and positive patterns of self-dialogue begin in early childhood. The patterns created at an early age can influence our thinking for most of our adult years. This can have a profound impact on us in many ways, particularly on the way stress can affect our lives. However, it is certainly possible to alter the pattern of this self-dialogue and in doing so you can stop negative self-dialogue from affecting your self-esteem and the way you deal with stress.

Awareness of your self-dialogue patterns

In order to alter a pattern we must first become aware of it. You are probably unaware of the level of negative self-dialogue that occurs in your head or how much it affects your life experience. The following approaches will enable you to become more aware of your internal self-dialogue.

Journaling – It can be useful to carry a notepad around with you, and whenever you become aware of a negative internal comment or dialogue, write it down. It is also useful at the end of the day to summarise your thoughts for the day with free flowing language. Later you can analyse this summary and you might begin to notice how negative tone or expressions creep into your language.

Replacing negative dialogue – An excellent method of improving your self-dialogue is to replace negative words with more positive or milder ones. You might have noticed how doctors will often use the word 'discomfort' rather than 'pain'. If you think about it, 'pain' has a much higher intensity and by using that word you are more likely to heighten the experience of pain rather experience the milder feeling of discomfort. You can use this approach when altering your own self-dialogue. Changing more powerful negative words to more neutral ones will usually help to neutralise your experience. Instead of using words like 'catastrophe' and 'disaster', you should use milder words such as 'challenge' and 'testing'. Here are some ideas for reducing word strength:

NEGATIVE WORD	MILDER ALTERNATIVE
Acute	Temporary
Aching	Niggling
Annoyed	Irked
Afraid	Uncomfortable
Alone	Waiting for Someone
Anxious	Restless
Chronic	Frequent
Disturbed	Moved
Exhausted	Gathering Energy
Failed	Moving Closer to Success
Frightened	Challenged
Helpless	Welcoming Support
Hopeless	Needing Encouragement

NEGATIVE WORD	MILDER ALTERNATIVE
Hurting	Uncomfortable
Lonely	Bored
Nervous	Expectant
Overwhelmed	In Demand
Out of Control	Making Changes
Painful	Uncomfortable
Scared	Eager
Sick	Recovering
Useless	Not required

Challenge your assumptions – If you find yourself mentally complaining about something, challenge your assumptions. Are you assuming something bad is going to happen even though it might not? If you find yourself worrying or stressing about something, stop and see if you can identify an alternative outcome that is neutral or even positive.

Alter self-limiting statements – Self-limiting statements are phrases like, I can't cope with this, or, This is impossible for me. These phrases are particularly unhelpful as they increase stress and can prevent you from finding solutions. If you notice yourself imposing limitations, turn the phrase into a question such as, How will I handle this?, or, How will I make this work? These phrases open your mind and imagination up to finding new solutions.

♀♂

THE FERTILITY CODE MIND PROGRAMME

You can help develop positive self-dialogue by following the Fertility Code Mind Programme that follows. This programme will help you to develop the optimum mind-frame for fertility and in doing so help to alleviate the effects of worry and stress.

Stage one

Reprogramming your mind for fertility

There is no set timeframe for this exercise. I would suggest giving yourself a number of weeks to slowly develop your ability.

Step one – Thought awareness

- Sit comfortably in a chair. Close your eyes and allow your body to relax and simply observe the flow of your thoughts for five minutes. Try to remember these thoughts. In the beginning you may notice that your thoughts relate to matters of everyday life; home- or work-related matters or worries may rush in on you. You must maintain the position of a silent observer, independently watching the flow of these thoughts. Depending on your state of mind, this exercise may be difficult or easy. If it seems difficult, try to maintain your train of thought and observe attentively.

- Start by practising this exercise twice a day, beginning for five minutes, and then each time you perform it, extend the duration by one minute until you are observing your thoughts for ten minutes without digression. Once finished, you should be able to recall the train of your thoughts for the duration of the exercise.

- As you practise, your thoughts will quickly become less chaotic. When you have mastered this exercise, your thoughts will become slow, ordered and easily remembered. At that stage you can move to step two.

Step two – Thought control: empowering a positive self-dialogue

☙ For the next stage of the exercise you will refuse to allow any negative self-dialogue to prevail in your thoughts. If any negative thought or statement such as, *I don't look good,* pops into your head, acknowledge the intent of the message, which in this case is that you want to look and feel good, and then immediately remove the negative statement from your mind.

☙ Collect the negative thought and imagine literally cleaning it out of your mind. Visualise yourself wiping it off a white board and say 'erase' in your head as you do so. Then replace the thought with a more positive equivalent such as, *I'm starting to feel good again.*

☙ If you find yourself slipping up, avoid self-criticism, as this simply compounds the issue. Move on and practise this exercise until you can comfortably follow your thoughts for ten minutes without allowing any negative thoughts to invade.

Step three – Thought mastery: the Seven-day Fertility Code Mind Reprogramme

You are now ready to move on to the final and most empowering stage of this exercise. You will learn how to retain a consistent state of mental positivity. By developing the habit of positivity you will become stronger, both mentally and physically.

☙ Over the next seven days refuse to dwell on any negative self-dialogue. This is to be practised throughout your day. You will reject all negative thoughts the instant they attack. Each such thought must be reframed and transformed from a negative thought into a positive thought, or else just rejected completely.

↪ When you find yourself focusing on any negative self-dialogue, immediately use the 'erase' method practised in step two. For these seven days you will train your mind to focus on positive solutions. As soon as you are confronted with a mental or physical challenge, immediately focus your attention on what you want the solution to be.

↪ If you slip up and find yourself dwelling on negative self-dialogue for any length of time, accept that you need to continue to work on this exercise and begin again from stage one. Because consistency is a key component of the exercise, it is important to begin at day one again if you do slip up. This will ensure that at the end of the seven days, your mind is re-patterned to consistently move towards positive self-dialogue and as a result the optimum mental framework for fertility.

♀ ♂

Stage two

The worry-dissolving Exercise

This exercise removes habitual worry and promotes a more positive and optimistic mental state.

Step one

Think for a moment about something that is currently worrying you. The nature of worry is that we contemplate a future event as if it has already happened. We imagine something going wrong, a poor result, not being able to cope with something, etc.

Step two

When you think about your worry, notice what images you create in your head, and any thoughts and feelings that manifest. You might not fully appreciate that you are creating these images and thoughts, but you are. Perhaps you might imagine, in full colour, receiving bad news and feel a knot in your stomach.

Step three

Now ask yourself if this worry helps you. If the answer is yes, then define how exactly it is useful. For example, in the case where you imagine an accident that might happen, you may take precautions so as to avoid it. If you are spending time worrying that something will not happen, as is often the case when people worry in relation to fertility, this might cause you to seek medical support, which could be helpful. It might also encourage you to support your fertility by following the Fertility Code. Once you have written down and acknowledged all the benefits of the worry, there is no longer any point in worrying. Some people might consider it beneficial to prepare mentally if things do not go as planned. However, being in a frequent state of turmoil and anxiety is never a good method of mental preparation.

Step four

Now imagine a visual of the worry being placed on a screen. You can now see the worry and hear the sounds as if it is happening on a film. Imagine placing this screen up and to your left.

Step five

Now imagine a future in which the thing you are worried about has actually happened. See yourself on another screen coping very well with this outcome. When observing this image, notice that you have also taken action as a result of step three in order to protect yourself. Because of this you see yourself smiling and looking calm and relaxed. Place this screen up and to your right.

Step six

Now, with your mind, imagine taking the screen with the original worry from the left and placing it right in front of you. Counting down – three, two, one – imagine the screen fading into the distance as the second screen (with the positive image) sweeps in and replaces the negative image. It is important to do this rapidly. Repeat this step five times or until the original worry is significantly diminished.

Stage 3

Prompt the Relaxation Response

We instinctively know how stress is having an effect on our body. Heart and breathing rates speed up, we have more muscular tension, our digestive system can play up and we can break into a sweat. This is the classic fight-or-flight response and the normal reaction when our brains anticipate that we are under threat. Ideally the stress ends when the threat ends, but in the modern world the perceived threat or danger is often ever-present. Unfortunately in this situation the stress reaction continues and can become chronic, never allowing our bodies to properly relax.

The Harvard cardiologist Dr Herbert Benson studied the affects of meditation on blood pressure and coined the term Relaxation Response. This is understood to be the countermeasure to the fight-or-flight response and allows homeostasis to occur. Homeostasis is where the body's systems return to a state of equilibrium. The Relaxation Response originates in the hypothalamus which, as we have already learned, is responsible for regulating the functions of the hormonal and nervous systems within your body. The connection between this hypothalamic reaction to stress and changes that take place in hormone secretion could have a role in many disorders associated with fertility. This is completely logical, for if your body is interpreting that you are under threat, it would make sense that it would interpret this as a bad time to become pregnant, and so it shuts down that function. For men, perhaps for this same reason, emotional stress is associated with abnormal sperm development.

Another hormone released in large quantities when you are under a lot of stress, be it physical or mental, is prolactin. When the pituitary gland releases this hormone it can lead to a lack of menstrual periods in women and can have an impact on sexual function in men.

The good news is that just as your body produces these hormonal reactions when experiencing stress, the Relaxation Response elicits the precise counterbalancing reaction necessary to restore hormonal balance.

The Relaxation Response involves creating a physical state of deep relaxation, which is triggered by a branch of the autonomic nervous system called the parasympathetic nervous system. The fight-or-flight response which was triggered by the sympathetic nervous system is switched off and your body and its biochemistry return to their pre-stress states.

Switching off the fight-or-flight response and switching on the Relaxation Response results in a decrease in heart rate, a lowering of blood pressure and a reduction in muscular tension. Your body effectively acknowledges that there is no longer a threat and the brain stops sending emergency signals to the brain stem, which in turn stops sending panic messages to the nervous system. Your physiology returns to pre-stress normality.

You can help this Relaxation Response to occur by listening to the Fertility Code Mind Programme CD which supports this book and is available on www.fertilitycode.com

You can also produce your own recording using the script below which guides you towards the Relaxation Response.

$$♀♂$$

Preparing for the guided Relaxation Response

1. A quiet place

Find a quiet place where you will be free from distractions. A bedroom is often suitable as it is a place where you should be used to resting. Having a quiet environment will make the exercise much easier to perform, as distracting thoughts are less likely to invade.

2. A point of focus

In everyday life we have constant stimulation and we are able to focus on more than one thing at a time. As you read this book you might also be aware of all the sounds around you. If there is too much external stimulation around you, your mind will wander from one thing to another. To prevent your mind wandering and to elicit the Relaxation Response you should create a single point of focus. This could be focusing your gaze on a single point like the flickering of a candle, or repeating a sound or word, either silently or out loud. This is called a mantra. If you choose to repeat the sound or word you should close your eyes. If you gaze at a single point, your eyes will remain open, of course. It can also be useful to bring your attention to the normal rhythm of your breathing.

3. Remaining passive

If you feel a distracting thought wandering in, simply allow it to pass by and direct your attention to the word repetition or the gaze. Be relaxed about how well you are performing this technique, as being concerned about it may in itself prevent the Relaxation Response from happening. Simply let it happen. This ability to remain passive is probably the most important element in eliciting the Relaxation Response. Distracting thoughts will occur but remain passive and they will fade. The fact that these thoughts are occurring does not mean you are practising the technique incorrectly as this is to be expected.

4. Comfortable posture

Maintaining a comfortable posture is important so as not to cause undue muscular tension. Some methods call for a sitting position. If you practise lying down, there is a tendency to fall asleep, so it is better to use a seated position. Whether you practise in a seated, standing or kneeling position you should be comfortable and relaxed.

The guided Relaxation Response

In this guided relaxation we are going to focus on a lighted candle.

- ✤ Locate a quiet place. Light a candle and sit in a comfortable position about three feet away from the flickering flame.

- ✤ Allow the focus of your eyes to soften as you gaze at the flame.

- ✤ Deeply relax all the muscles in your body, beginning at your toes, then move to your feet, ankles, legs, lower back, fingers, hands, shoulders, neck and progress up your face to the top of your head. Stay relaxed.

- ✤ Breathe softly through your nose. Become aware of your breathing. As you breathe maintain your gaze on the flickering candle. It is perfectly fine to blink. Breathe slowly and naturally.

- ✤ Continue this for approximately fifteen minutes, but do not use an alarm. The time does not have to be exact. When you are finished, sit quietly for several minutes. Allow your eyes to open fully. Stay sitting for a few minutes before you stand.

- ✤ Be comfortable with the amount of deep relaxation you have achieved. Maintain a passive attitude and relaxation will occur at its own pace. If distracting thoughts do occur, remain passive and allow them to drift by.

- ✤ With practice, the Relaxation Response will come with very little effort. Practise this technique twice daily initially. Don't practise after meals, as the digestive processes can interfere with your ability to elicit the Relaxation Response.

Stage 4

Progressive Muscle Relaxation

Progressive Muscle Relaxation (PMR) is a simple but powerful stress management technique developed by the American physician Edmund Jacobson in the early 1920s. Jacobson recognised that there was a link between muscular tension and stress and he believed that as muscular tension generally accompanies stress, if it was possible to reduce this muscular tension it would by default reduce the stress effect on your body. By guiding his patients to consciously and purposefully relax the muscles in their bodies, he was able to reduce their stress-related symptoms. This technique was found to be effective at treating a number of stress related conditions such as depression, anxiety, irritable bowel syndrome, back pain and hypertension.

Progressive Muscle Relaxation may be practised lying on your back or sitting in a chair with your head supported. As you begin practising you might find that you only partially relax, but with time and practice you can use this technique to achieve deep levels of relaxation in just a few minutes.

How to practise Progressive Muscle Relaxation

- Lie on your back with your eyes closed, feet slightly apart and arms slightly away from your sides with palms facing upwards.

- Allow your breathing to slow. Turn your attention now to your breath. Notice as you draw it in and out. Pause to become aware of this for twenty seconds.

- Tense the muscles in your feet for five seconds, then gently allow them to relax. Pause in the relaxed state for twenty seconds, then repeat.

- Next tense the muscles of your calves for five seconds, then relax and allow all the tension in your lower legs to drift away. Pause for twenty seconds and repeat.

♘ Next tense the muscles in your thighs for five seconds, then relax and let this tension go. Pause in this relaxed state for twenty seconds and repeat.

♘ Now tense the muscles in your abdomen for five seconds, then relax and let this tension go. Pause in this relaxed state for twenty seconds and repeat.

♘ Now move to your chest. Tense your chest muscles for five seconds. Relax for twenty seconds and repeat.

♘ Clench your fists really tightly for five seconds, then relax your hands completely and let the tension drift away for twenty seconds and repeat.

♘ Next flex your elbows and tense your biceps. Hold your upper arm bicep muscles really tight for five seconds then relax and straighten your arms. Feel this relaxation for twenty seconds and repeat.

♘ Tense the muscles of your neck for five seconds. Relax. Let the tension go and pause for twenty seconds, then repeat.

♘ Finally tense the muscles of your head and face for five seconds. Allow your facial expression to tense up completely for these five seconds before letting all this tightness drift away for twenty seconds. Then repeat.

♀♂

Stage 5

Enhancing sleep

There seems to be quite a lot of confusion about the importance of sleep. There are many self-help books on the market that promise greater productivity by reducing the amount of time you spend sleeping. There are well-known historical figures, such as

Margaret Thatcher, Winston Churchill, Bill Clinton and Napoleon Bonaparte, who survived on very little sleep. However, the fact that they were world leaders doesn't mean that they experienced good health. Napoleon famously said, 'Six for the man, seven for the woman and eight for the fool,' when he referred to how much sleep should be taken. But it is also worth noting that Napoleon had a host of ailments, which included depression, epilepsy, scabies, neurodermatitis, migraine, chronic hepatitis and stomach cancer. He was also just fifty-one when he died. So I believe that this opinion that we do not need much sleep to function well and maintain good health is completely flawed. Napoleon was certainly a great general, but he probably wasn't someone I would have gone to for healthy lifestyle advice.

In relation to fertility, there is a growing opinion that adequate sleep is a vital factor in improving your chances of conception. When we achieve good quality sleep, our bodies repair cells and regulate our hormones, among many other processes. One important hormone, leptin, is an important link between fertility and sleep. Leptin is critical for ovulation, and women need adequate sleep in order to produce adequate leptin. If leptin production is compromised, menstrual cycles are frequently disrupted.

Sleep also affects the production of other key fertility hormones including progesterone, oestrogen, luteinising hormone (LH) and follicle stimulating hormone (FSH). Research shows that as much as 90 per cent of ovulation occurs between midnight and 4 a.m. If you are sleep-deprived, your body will focus on preserving critical functions, like strengthening your immune system, rather than conception. We know that a lack of sleep disrupts our circadian rhythm, the twenty-four-hour internal clock that helps regulate our body's systems.

Why are you sleep deprived?

People are sleep-deprived for three reasons. First of all, for some people it is because their job requires them to work night shifts. Research has shown that people who work at night have a much harder time getting pregnant. Women who work at night have a much greater tendency to have irregular menstrual cycles. Being in tune with nature by sleeping when it is nighttime and being awake during the day helps our circadian rhythm to function normally.

A second reason that people are sleep-deprived is habit. Many people are working longer hours, and because they get home late at night, they resist going to bed early as they feel they are depriving themselves of recreation and wind-down time. Whilst this is understandable, if it is having an impact on the amount of sleep you are getting, it is not helpful.

The third reason that people are sleep-deprived is that they suffer with insomnia. This can manifest in a number of ways. For some people their minds are too active and they have difficulty falling asleep. Others have no difficulty falling asleep but frequently wake up during the night and have difficulty falling back asleep. Yet others will fall asleep and stay asleep, but never get to the deeper levels of unconsciousness required for our bodies to fully recover. These people will often spend much of the night in the dream state and when morning comes they may even feel exhausted from their dreams.

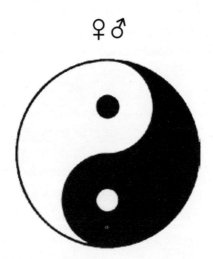

Balancing yin and yang

You have probably seen this symbol many times. This is called the yin yang symbol and it comes from the Chinese Taoist philosophy. The literal translation of yin is 'the dark side of the hill' and yang is 'the sunny side of the hill'. What this symbol really represents is balance and also the interdependence of the opposing forces in nature and the universe. Yin represents everything that is cooling, nourishing, moistening and quiet, and yang represents everything that is warming, drying and activating. Yin represents nighttime, autumn and winter, when it is quieter and cooler, and yang represents daytime, spring and summer, when there is more activity and, typically, it is warmer. This symbol can be seen to represent the cycles of life and of nature and within Chinese medicine the yin yang theory is a central concept. In terms of sleep, what this theory tells us is that we should be in tune with nature. We should therefore sleep at night and be active during the day. Chinese medicine would also tell us that during autumn and winter we need more sleep than in spring and summer.

In relation to the first two causes of sleep deprivation there isn't much to say. If you work nights and there is an option for you to work fewer night shifts, then this is something you should try to do. If you are in the habit of staying up late at night rather than going to bed early, take action and break that habit in order to get at least eight hours' sleep every night. You will soon feel the benefits.

For anyone dealing with any of the forms of insomnia mentioned, here are a few suggestions that should help you to achieve better sleep.

Follow a set routine

Develop a set pattern before bed that allows you to clear your mind. Go through the same patterns each night. This might be brushing your hair, cleaning your face, brushing your teeth, kissing your partner good night. All of these within a wind-down pattern can help settle you down in preparation for sleep. We will look at coffee later and generally discourage its intake, but before bed it is particularly unhelpful to consume any drinks containing caffeine. If you do take caffeine, try to restrict it to before noon each day, after you wake in the mornings. If you need to drink before bedtime, consider a soothing mug of camomile tea, which is more conducive to sleep. Avoid having too much to drink before bedtime, however, or your sleep may be interrupted by the need to go to the bathroom.

Create the right setting

You should ensure that your bedroom is conducive to sleep. Remove all the clutter and make sure that your bed and pillow are comfortable. Make sure that you have clean sheets. It is also a good idea not to overstimulate your brain before attempting to fall asleep. This means switching off the TV at least twenty minutes before retiring. If you read in bed, make sure you give yourself some time to wind down after you finish reading.

Soothing colours may also help you to fall asleep faster than bright, vibrant colours. Research has shown that colours affect mood, and light, natural colours generally elicit a greater sense of calm than vibrant colours. It is a good idea to keep the lights dim in the bedroom and keep the temperature at around 21°C.

I would also suggest that you keep a notebook and pen beside your bed. If your mind is too active, writing down the issues you are thinking about should help you to park them until the morning.

Exercise for sleep

Exercise makes falling asleep and staying asleep easier. Later on in the evening, prior to bed, it is better for your exercise to be of a slow nature. This helps to prepare both body and mind for sleep. Chi kung (or qigong) is an ancient Chinese exercise system performed to calm the mind and is therefore an ideal exercise for relaxation prior to bed. Chi Kung loosely translates as energy training. The system joins movement and breathing with intent, which can produce considerable stress reduction benefits.

Finding a way to achieve a restful sleep every night can take time. It is important to get the basics right and to think of optimising your sleep as a key part of what you are doing to prepare for pregnancy.

♀♂

Stage 6

Meditation

Meditation is widely acknowledged as one of the most effective ways to improve your response to stress. Meditation is practised throughout the globe by millions of people. Those who do not meditate often mistakenly believe that it is too complex and too difficult to do. Like many things, however, meditation is simply a skill that takes a bit of learning.

Meditation is a central element of the Fertility Code Mind Programme. You should integrate it into your life and use it often. As you develop your meditation skills, you will find that it improves your clarity of thought and your decision-making ability. It also helps you to organise your thoughts and, consequently, handle stress better.

How meditation works

Meditation is easy, but as with many skills you need to learn how to do it properly. The first surprise for many is just how undisciplined your mind really is and how easily it can be distracted. Try this simple test. Set an alarm for five minutes from now and count each breath you take until then, without thinking of anything else. It's not an easy task. One of the main objectives of meditation is to train your mind to focus on what you choose. As part of this goal, with practice, you learn how to empty your mind of thought.

When you learn to empty your mind you will free yourself from the stresses of daily life that prevent your mind from finding peace, sometimes even when you are asleep. If you empty your mind, you no longer experience stress in that moment and where stress has a physical dimension, this also starts to fade away.

How meditation can benefit your fertility

Meditation produces a deep state of physiological relaxation, decreases your heart rate, lowers your metabolic rate (the rate at which you expend energy), improves your digestion and causes an overall sense of relaxation. This slower metabolism combined with lower heart rate means that less oxygen is required and consequently you produce less carbon dioxide. This lowers the concentration of lactic acid in the blood, which at high levels is associated with anxiety and stress. Studies have shown that the lactic acid levels in the blood of people who regularly meditate are just a quarter of those of the average person who doesn't meditate.

Meditation creates a state of rest and physical renewal. Your muscles relax and your food is digested properly. The heart rate slows and blood circulation to the body's tissues increases, feeding your body with nutrients and oxygen. This restful state achieved through meditation is good for your fertility as it allows your body to conserve the resources it needs to generate a new life.

Preparing for meditation

Stage one of the Fertility Code Mind Programme – Reprogramme your Mind for Fertility – is an excellent way to prepare your mind for meditation. This exercise helps you to become more aware of your thoughts and more in control of directing your thoughts.

The key to meditation for fertility is to focus on one relaxing thought for a sustained period of time. This calms your mind and gives your body the chance to relax and recuperate. This clears away toxic thoughts that may have built up through stress and mental activity.

The essence of meditation is to quiet your thoughts by focusing completely on one thing. Hypnotic trance is somewhat similar, though often a passive experience. Meditation is an active process that aims to exclude outside thoughts by concentrating your full focus on the meditation subject.

Meditation should be performed in a position that you can comfortably remain in for a period of time, ideally twenty minutes or so. Sitting on a comfortable chair is effective, but in certain circumstances you can even meditate when walking.

The preparations we did for Stage 3, Prompt the Relaxation Response, and Stage 4, Progressive Muscle Relaxation, also build towards excellent meditation practice. The following are some further important elements for meditation practice:

↳ Set aside time to meditate. Make some time available every day to meditate. The effects of meditation are cumulative and are far more significant if you practise regularly and consistently rather than occasionally for longer periods.

You can practise at any time of the day, but I think morning meditation provides an ideal start to the day. You may also like to meditate at the end of the day, as it is good practice to clear your mind before going to sleep. For those who have stressful jobs, meditating at lunchtime in the middle of the day can provide a mental sanctuary from the chaos of a busy day. Generally, however, I think it is easier to meditate in the morning, before the day's events tire you out.

↳ Meditate in a quiet, relaxing place. As with some of the previous exercises, when you are practising meditation it is important to avoid distractions. Switch off your TV, phone, radio and anything else that may cause distraction. If you like to meditate to music, use sounds that are calm, repetitive and gentle, without vocals.

↳ Find a comfortable posture. It is important to feel physically relaxed when meditating, as any discomfort can in itself cause distraction. You do not have to twist legs into a lotus position or adopt any unusual postures. These postures are uncomfortable for most people and are not helpful for beginners. It is however good to keep your back straight as this can help with breathing.

↳ Relax the muscles in your body. Take your time to relax. The Progressive Muscle Relaxation exercise is a really good way to prepare your body for meditation. Perform this exercise then breathe out, letting all your muscles go at once. Feel yourself letting go of all your tension. Enjoy the feeling of relaxation as your muscles let go more and more.

✤ Focus your attention. If your mind wishes to wander, moving from thought to thought, gently guide it back to a single point until it rests there naturally. The goal is to allow the 'chattering' in your mind to gradually fade away. The earlier exercises in the Fertility Mind Programme should help you to achieve this.

Another useful approach is to allow your attention to focus on your breath. Listen to it, notice it and follow it, without making any comments about it. Simply count your breaths from one to ten and then start again at one.

To prevent the intrusion of distracting mental images, visualise a place that calms you. This can be a real place or an imagined one. You could imagine descending a staircase that leads you deeper and deeper into tranquillity.

✤ Quiet your mind. Once you have trained your mind to focus on just one thing at a time, you can practise the next step, which is to focus on nothing at all. Essentially this means clearing your mind. After spending a while focusing on a single point, such as your breath, you can allow it to drift away without labelling it or making any internal comments. Follow the same approach with any thoughts that return to your mind, until you achieve a sustained silence. This is meditation.

Guided meditation

Guided meditation is a technique in which the person is led through the meditative process by a soothing voice which can help you to achieve a state of peacefulness and clarity. In many cases, hypnotic techniques are used, which can be helpful in deepening the meditative state. The calming voice may also include language that helps to conjure up images to increase a sense of inner calm and support meditation.

Guided meditation is particularly helpful for anyone who is

beginning their meditative practice. The Fertility Code Mind Programme CD includes a powerful guided meditation. You could also record and play back, or have someone slowly read, the following script in a soft pitch and tone.

The idea is that you allow your conscious mind to switch off while following the words that are being spoken on a subconscious level. What many people like about guided meditation is that they can effortlessly achieve a deep state of relaxation whilst still retaining subconscious awareness.

Guided fertility meditation script

- ⌗ Begin by sitting comfortably with your back supported. Allow your body to relax. Your feet are touching the ground, with your arms relaxed on your lap. Take a deep breath in and let all tension go. Now notice your breathing. Notice how steady it is – first in ... then out. As you breathe in, visualise clean, white energy filling your lungs. Then, as you breathe out, feel any toxins or stress exit your body as grey mist.

- ⌗ Breathe in the white and breathe out the grey, keeping the same slow but steady pace. Focus on the increased feeling of relaxation and vitality for ten deep inhalations and ten full exhalations. Notice the energy that is in your body and notice the sensations of warmth and comfort that begin to permeate each cell and fibre in your body. Notice the sensations of the energy around you on the surface of your skin. As you relax more deeply, feel the external energies and internal energies blend together.

- ⌗ Now visualise warm, soothing energy shining down from above your head. Bring this shining, glowing energy down through the top of your head and feel it melting like warm oil, down into your body. Feel it melt relaxation and healing down the front of your face, your neck, shoulders, and down into your arms. Feel this healing energy melting through every cell in your body, down your chest, into your abdomen, and washing all over your reproductive system, before settling on your legs to your toes.

♺ Notice that your whole body is filled with healing light and energy, and observe that your legs and body feel lighter. Allow this healing energy to completely fill your physical space with a deep sense of relaxation. You may want to smile as you feel a warm glowing sensation all over your body. Let this sensation go deeper and deeper into the core of your body. Sit in this golden light and focus on your slow breathing. Keep focusing your breathing as you begin to count down from ten. Ten ... nine ... eight ... seven ... six ... slowly start to wiggle your fingers and toes ... five ... four ... gradually lift and stretch your arms ... three ... two ... one ... open your eyes, feeling bright and alert; feeling great!

Practise this guided meditation regularly and you will feel more relaxed and will notice that you cope better with life's stresses. This in turn will enhance your immunity, increase your sense of well-being and in turn improve your fertility. When you consider the amount of time you have spent stressing and worrying in the past, it seems reasonable to now allow yourself to enjoy greater and deeper relaxation. This guided meditation is an efficient way to help you achieve this.

♀♂

CHAPTER SUMMARY

As you've probably realised, it is impossible to completely avoid stress. Stress is a necessary part of life and in some cases it can be helpful, for example when you need extra adrenaline in times of danger. Stress, however, does not have to be a negative issue provided that you know how to deal with it in the correct manner.

The stress management methods covered in this chapter build

towards a daily routine and are a key element of the Fertility Code. A successful stress management programme will also include elements from the rest of the Fertility Code, including proper nutrition, appropriate exercise and detoxification.

- ♮ You have learned some powerful ways to manage your own brain. When you practise these exercises you can change the way the "software" in your brain works and bring benefits to the way you feel physically and emotionally. Embracing the Fertility Code Mind Programme should not only benefit your health, but also enhance the quality of your life and improve your fertility.

- ♮ Indulge in constant mental positivity. Continue to work through this book, but return to this chapter and continue to practise the mind programming exercises in this chapter. By performing the exercises you create the mental foundation for improved health and fertility.

- ♮ You should aim to incorporate thirty minutes of The Fertility Code Mind Programme into your daily routine. This will move you towards an effective way to better manage stress. The key is persistence and discipline. If dedicating thirty minutes daily seems like it may cause time pressure, then that is probably a fair indication that you definitely need to use the Fertility Code Mind Programme!

- ♮ The Fertility Code Mind Program CD is available from **www.fertilitycode.com;** the CD supports this chapter and guides you through many of the techniques.

- ♮ Probably the most important lesson from this chapter is that you are responsible for the manner in which your mind operates. From here on you should seize this control.

♀♂

A Cognitive BEHAVIOURAL Approach

ANN BRACKEN

Fertility Counselling Psychotherapist,
Sims IVF Clinic

INTRODUCTION

The emotional and psychological well-being of couples and individuals who undergo fertility treatment is very important. Supporting the psychological, emotional and physical well-being of both women and men experiencing fertility issues has been shown to positively affect fertility. According to Dr Alice Domar, who pioneered the Mind/Body Programme at Harvard University, 'Several studies conducted within the past three years support the theory that psychological distress can have a significant adverse impact on success rates in in vitro fertilisation (IVF). Mind/body treatment of infertility patients has been shown to both increase pregnancy rates as well as reduce psychological distress.'

Facing infertility issues is one of the most challenging experiences an individual or couple can go through. Before seeking fertility support treatment (either natural health or medically assisted), most individuals have already gone through a range of thoughts and feelings, either in response to their own beliefs or those of others, such as family and friends. The experience can trigger some powerful negative emotions, including low mood/depression, grief, anxiety, anger, unhealthy envy, loss of self-esteem, feelings of being judged harshly by others, and guilt.

Integrating stress-reduction techniques and establishing self-supportive thinking patterns and beliefs can improve your well-being by encouraging self-acceptance and compassion in the face of a deeply personal or couple crisis. This can bring about a positive change in your overall health, ease relationship problems and improve your emotional experience.

HOW CAN COGNITIVE BEHAVIOURAL THERAPY HELP?

Cognitive behavioural therapy (CBT) works on the understanding that there is a correlation between our internal dialogue and our corresponding emotions. It essentially aims to change the way we feel by challenging and changing unhelpful thoughts and beliefs about our experiences. Firstly, it is helpful to understand the types of thoughts or beliefs you hold about your experience of dealing with infertility.

Unhelpful thoughts that may arise when feeling stressed with issues relating to fertility

- This has to work or it means I'm a failure (self-downing)

- If it wasn't for me, my partner would have a better life (fortune telling with negative filter)

- Everyone else has it easy (over-generalising)

- My life is not worth living unless I can have a baby (life-negating and discounting your positive qualities and worth)

- People absolutely shouldn't ask me if I want a baby (other-downing even if they are unaware of your challenges)

- Others are doing much better than me (over-generalising)

- Other women drink and smoke and still give birth – life shouldn't be like this (black-and-white thinking; things should be absolute, in black or white categories)

- I left it too late (over-personalising responsibility, as the individual/couple were not aware that they had an issue; lacks compassion)

♀ It's his/her fault or it's my fault (personalisation and blame – you blame yourself/other for something/medical issue that you are not responsible for).

♀♂

Whilst it is completely understandable to have negative feelings relating to the crisis that may be associated with infertility, if we leave unhelpful thinking unchallenged, it can deepen the crisis by triggering emotions that are hard to manage (e.g. anxiety and/or anger). Often our negative thoughts about ourselves and our partner are untrue and cruel. However, these thoughts have a huge emotional impact. We may attach our struggle with fertility treatment with a self-downing lie, e.g. if this doesn't work, people will judge me/us and it will mean I'm a failure. This unhelpful and harsh interpretation of a perceived future can fuel further negative thoughts and this can affect our behaviour, perhaps causing us to avoid others or push our partner away and sabotage the relationship because we believe 'they would be better without me'. In addition, unhelpful thinking styles can lead to sleep disturbance, irritability, or an inability to settle (constantly busy, rushing around and seeking reassurance from others regularly).

When you notice your negative automatic thoughts (NATS), take a breath before you respond; don't react automatically. Exploring the nature of these thoughts in a journal can help us access our deepest beliefs. Understanding what motivates our harsh thinking styles can prompt us to change them and, in so doing, to become compassionate towards ourselves and others. This awareness also affects the choices we make when facing a stressful situation.

The following exercise aims to support you in understanding your negative thinking patterns and encourages you to replace them with more self-supportive thoughts and actions.

Write down your most unhelpful thoughts and ask yourself:

- Is this thought true?
- Is it absolutely true about me/him?
- Is this a belief I have had about myself in other situations?
- If so, where and when did I learn it? (Usually from an early life experience.)
- Prove it. Write down the evidence that this thought is true.
- Disprove it. Write down the evidence that does not support this thought.
- Do I believe that I will be judged harshly by others? Is that likely? Everybody?
- What would happen if I let go of thinking about myself in this way?
- What would I tell my best friend if she had this thought in this situation?
- Am I underestimating my ability to cope in difficult situations?

(List some life challenging events you have coped with in the past.)

- What supportive resources (people, places, things) do I have?
- How do my reactions affect me?
- How do they affect others?
- Is there anything I can change about this situation, my environment, my reaction, or my behaviour right now?
- Is this situation within my control or out of my control?
- If the current situation is out of my control, can I make an action plan or a plan B?

- Can I re-focus my attention to, for example, some soothing music, a safe place, a comforting friend or a plan of action, to support me in the present moment-to-moment managing of stress?
- Do I believe that I am only of value if I have a baby?
- Would I believe this of another woman/man? Why not?
- Is there a different way to perceive this situation, or to perceive myself/my partner in this situation?
- Identify your stressors – the part of the process that you become most stressed about – and establish coping techniques for those times.

The following coping statements will help support you through the various stages of treatment:

- I/we are doing everything in our power to support myself/ourselves in my/our desire to have a baby, which takes great courage.

- I've gone through this procedure before and I can do it now.

- This part of the process (e.g. taking medication or tolerating needles) will pass. It is only temporary.

- Keep going; it is worth it to me to go through this discomfort to achieve my long-term goal

- I am a worthwhile person.

- I can make wise decisions based on what I know.

- I am a strong woman/man.

- This isn't comfortable or pleasant but I can manage it.

- Resisting this isn't going to help me; I can breathe and accept myself through this challenge.

Dealing with grief

Understanding why we are feeling difficult emotions can help us achieve the acceptance we need to move through those emotions and not become stuck in the discomfort. For example, many individuals and couples go through a cycle of grief when they are told they have fertilty issues. This can also happen if a couple experience a negative outcome. This cycle varies in intensity and duration and each partner may experience it to a different extent. Even in a shared experience, we are all unique in how we process loss or disappointment.

Elizabeth Kubler Ross first outlined the stages experienced by people overcoming loss and bereavement. This cycle of grief and loss may include:

- Shock and disorganisation – this can also be experienced as a sense that time is standing still. Patients have also expressed this as a feeling of being 'numbed' or having an out-of-body experience.

- Protest – this usually involves undertaking practical tasks or avoidance strategies in an attempt to distance ourselves from intense feelings of loss.

- Bargaining and what ifs – naturally, we aim to bring some understanding to a profoundly difficult experience and may constantly replay small details relating to the event in the hope of changing it.

- Following a bereavement you may experience low mood/depression for a time.

- Acceptance – we finally experience a sense of acceptance that the situation is as it is.

- Organisation – with acceptance we can then begin to establish an alternative plan to support ourselves moving forward.

- Not all individuals experience loss in the same way. Within a couple, one person may experience all the stages of grief whereas their partner may experience some of the stages and to a lesser extent. This can be difficult for both partners. The important thing is to accept your feelings and work through them.

Self-supportive plan

It can be helpful to establish a self-supportive plan as we can only draw water from a well with water in it. Making time to nurture yourself and your relationship ensures that you have the resources to optimise fertility and increase your confidence as you go through a treatment process. Having a sense of closeness to ourselves and others also increases self-acceptance and personal fulfilment.

Self-nurturing support can include:

- Relaxation techniques. Find one that works for you and aim to practise it three times a day.

- Compile a relaxation CD of your favourite music. You may also wish to listen to this when undergoing medical procedures, such as scans, transfers etc.

- If you meditate, allocate a time each day dedicated to this activity.

- Mindful activity. Focus your attention fully on another activity.

- Be with others. Contact a supportive friend or an understanding family member.

- Do something different. Observe how you respond when challenged and try to modify your response and learn a more helpful approach.

- Grounding techniques. Often we can become caught up in our internal world and self-dialogue, and we become disassociated with the reality of our here-and-now experience. Turn off your automatic pilot and divert your focus to your environment, taking it in with all your senses. What do you see, hear, smell, taste and feel? Think of an imaginary safe place that

you enjoy and take yourself there by visualising it.
Draw on this visualisation to prompt a relaxation
response.

༕ Hold a comforting object or a favourite picture/
photograph before going through a procedure.

༕ Learn to communicate assertively (rather than
passively or aggressively) and write down your
questions for your medical practitioner or doctor.

༕ Engage in a hobby or other interest. What have you
enjoyed in the past, before you became aware of
fertility issues? Remember that fertility issues are not
100 per cent of who you are.

༕ Learn some mindfulness-based relaxation techniques
such as breath work, body scan or mindful movement
(e.g. gentle low impact yoga) as they elicit a deep
relaxation response, balancing hormones and
releasing endorphins, to positively influence your
mood.

♀♂

Try these mini mindfulness-based relaxation techniques to help
restore balance before, during or after facing a medical procedure
or intervention.

Breathwork exercise

Breathe in through your nose, taking a deep breath in and down into
your abdominal area. Place your hand on the abdominal area, which
should rise and fall with each in and out breath. Position your lips
as though breathing through a straw. Close your eyes and breathe in
through your nose and breathe out through your lips. Become aware
of the breath on the inhale. Notice how it feels in your nostrils and
on the back of your throat, and follow the breath into the abdominal
area. In your mind, with each in breath, say 'in' and with each out
breath say 'out' or 'letting go'. Breathe in slowly through the nose
and exhale, letting go on the out breath (your mouth shaped as an

O). As you continue to breathe mindfully, you may notice that you have drifted into your thoughts and what they mean (Should I do this? Am I doing this right? Should I be somewhere else? etc.). Just notice that your mind has wandered and gently take your focus back to your breath again. You may also notice that your attention is drawn to a sensation or feeling in your body. Again, notice this and take your focus gently back to your breath. Continue this until you feel relaxed, and then continue some more!

Safe-place exercise

Imagine you are in your safe place, a favourite place where you feel completely relaxed. The safe place can be real or imaginary. Go to your safe place in your imagination, alone, and find comfort. Ask yourself what you can hear in your safe place (perhaps a brook, or leaves rustling in a wood), what would you expect to see in your safe place and what do you smell there? Connect to how you feel (calm) and where you feel it (e.g. in the chest area). Bring yourself to your safe place through your senses and keep breathing – deeply in through your nose and out through your mouth – as you take yourself there. Give your safe place a name, and when you feel stressed, just remind yourself to take yourself there. You can take yourself to your safe place lying down or sitting up with your eyes closed.

♀♂

If you notice that your negative feelings are not diminishing and that they are becoming more challenging, you may benefit from fertility counselling support or from visiting a medical practitioner. Counselling and psychotherapy can provide you with a source of emotional support and psychological insight in addition to providing you with mental health resource materials.

♀♂

THE
Fertility CODE
Nutrition Plan

"He who takes medicine and neglects diet wastes the skills of the physician"

Chinese proverb

INTRODUCTION

The Fertility Code Nutrition Plan can dramatically improve your fertility. The plan is very similar to an eating plan you would follow to maximise your general health. This makes perfect sense, of course: if your body is nourished properly, it follows that it will also be better prepared to nourish and produce a baby. I purposely call this a nutrition plan as opposed to a diet plan because the word diet has connotations of a weight-loss goal and the objective of our nutrition plan is not weight loss, but rather enhanced fertility. That being said, being overweight does have a detrimental effect on fertility for both men and women. In fact when both parties are overweight they are three times more likely to have fertility problems compared with couples of healthy weight. Being just 10 per cent over or under your ideal body weight can affect your fertility. By implementing the Fertility Code Nutrition Plan, your calorie intake is likely to be optimal. This means that if you are already at your ideal weight and you follow this plan you will not lose weight. However, it is also true that if you are overweight, you will inevitably lose weight if you follow the plan.

Case study – Claire and James

This case details the very frequent and often puzzling scenario – secondary infertility. This is when a couple have difficulty conceiving after they have already successfully had a baby. This case illustrates how Eastern medicine's common-sense approach can sometimes make all the difference and offers a rational explanation for such 'unexplainable' incidences of infertility.

Claire (32) and James (34) already had their little boy Mark together, with no other pregnancies. They successfully conceived within a very short timeframe and when Mark was approaching his first birthday they decided that they would like to try for another baby. They assumed that things would happen quite quickly for them. However, by the time Mark was five years old they had endured four years of unsuccessful attempts to conceive naturally. They then decided to visit a fertility clinic, where Claire had a laparoscopy and abdominal ultrasound. Based on the tests the doctor determined that there was no physical impediment to her conceiving. This was followed by tests on James that likewise showed no reason why conception had not occurred. Although there were no male or female factor issues found, Claire and James were very distressed. Without a physical factor to deal with, there was no opportunity to address the problem. They decided to work with the assistance of the fertility clinic and Claire began taking the ovarian stimulation drug, Clomid, and had a total of three unsuccessful intrauterine insemination (IUI) procedures. The fertility clinic then suggested that Claire and James should see me in preparation for a fourth IUI procedure.

Claire was extremely discouraged by all of this, and when she came to my clinic she said she felt so desperately down about it all that she now believed she was depressed. During our consultation it became clear that there were also times in the past when Claire had felt quite down. In fact shortly after Mark was born she had been prescribed a mild antidepressant when she had experienced an extended period of feeling low. Although Claire's pregnancy had been quite comfortable, the birth itself had been difficult. Due to complications Claire had to undergo an emergency Caesarean section, during which she lost quite a lot of blood. They felt that all was well in the end, however, and they were relieved to welcome Mark who was born healthy and well.

Apart from feeling down, Claire felt that she was physically well and had no significant health problems. However, on closer reflection there were many signs that things were not as well as they had been before Mark was conceived. After Mark's birth Claire had found it very difficult to sleep. This is quite natural when you have a newborn, but now years later she still experienced significant sleep problems. Although she could fall asleep, she almost always woke during the night and found it very difficult to fall back to sleep.

When the time came to get up in the morning, she always felt exhausted.

Along with this there were other issues, none of which Claire felt merited a visit to the doctor. Claire frequently felt bouts of extremely low energy, which as a working mum she had put down to being busier than she was before. She was also much more prone to colds and her circulation was poorer than it had been before. She suffered regular dizzy spells, fairly frequent headaches and she also noticed that her nails had become very brittle. More recently she had developed mild eczema.

The Chinese medical view

Chinese medicine understands that during the postnatal period mothers are vulnerable and prone to becoming depleted. This can result in developing what is called blood and/or energy deficiency (xue or qi xu). During this time women are advised to focus for one hundred days on nourishment, with the aim of rebuilding their energy. The lifestyle advice given during this time is to regularly eat highly nourishing foods and to get as much rest as possible. Exercise and work should be limited to help the woman recover fully from the birth. This process is frequently referred to as 'mother warming' in Chinese medical traditions.

Claire had not given such focus to her recovery when Mark was born. Now over five years later she still had legacy symptoms. In preparation for their fourth IUI she embarked on a Fertility Code Nutrition Plan, designed to nourish her back to full health and well-being. Claire flourished on the plan, so much so that she and James cancelled the IUI when after just three months they conceived naturally. Nine months later they welcomed Ava, a healthy baby girl, into their family.

♀♂

THE FERTILITY CODE NUTRITION PLAN

KEY PRINCIPLES

1. Eat large quantities of organic fruit and vegetables.

2. Replace bad fats with good fats.

3. Eat hormone-balancing phytoestrogens, such as beans, lentils and chickpeas daily

4. Eat healthy sources of lean protein

5. Eliminate dairy products

6. Avoid refined carbohydrates, including sugar, white bread and pasta

7. Avoid additives, preservatives and chemicals, such as artificial sweeteners and flavours

8. Drink at least two litres of water a day and restrict alcohol consumption to two units per week

9. Replace coffee or tea with green or jasmine tea

10. Replace refined table salt with healthy spices

Changing your eating habits

Changing from poor or even average eating habits to optimum nutrition is probably the most powerful thing you can do to enhance your fertility. By getting your nutrition right you will make a significant step towards preparing your body for conception and a healthy pregnancy. You will help yourself to sustain balanced blood sugar levels, regulate hormone levels, improve your digestion and achieve a healthy weight. Nutrition is key to the Fertility Code.

Although there is no miracle food that can suddenly make pregnancy occur, there are many foods that I recommend because of the overall benefits they deliver to your health, well-being and ultimately to your fertility. When you enjoy a balanced diet that includes plenty of nutrient-rich fruit and vegetables, you will feel better within yourself and more positive about the increased fertility you are working towards. It is important to note that this nutrition plan is not all about restricting calorie intake and you should always make sure to eat regularly throughout the day, as long as you're eating the right kind of food.

The key is to make healthy eating a part of your everyday life. Good nutrition has a subtle but powerful effect on your body over time. When I changed my own diet it took a few weeks for me to feel the full benefits. But by sustaining good eating habits, these benefits can be permanent and it is only by sticking with them that you will realise the long-term benefits of improved health and increased fertility.

Weight control

For many people the food they eat represents more than just a source of nutrition. Food can be a source of emotional comfort, a means of socialising and it is a central part of family life. Moreover, despite much media attention on the importance of healthy eating, obesity, fast-food consumption and eating disorders are all on the increase. The chances of conceiving and having a healthy pregnancy are significantly greater if both members of a couple are close to their ideal weight. For a woman, being overweight can cause abnormal menstrual cycles, which can lead to infertility. Overweight women are more likely to encounter pregnancy complications, such as hypertension and diabetes, and also have more difficult deliveries. It is estimated that up to 12 per cent of female fertility-related problems are directly linked to body weight (van der Steeg, 2008). Interestingly this is divided evenly between women who are overweight and women who are underweight, both being twice as likely to experience fertility problems. Overweight men also encounter fertility problems more frequently. A low sperm count correlates with being overweight, and overweight men have lower than average testosterone levels. As weight increases testosterone can be converted to oestrogen, which in turn can impair sperm production.

Another large-scale research project, The Harvard Nurses' Health Study, also found that overweight women took on average twice as long to get pregnant, but it found that underweight women took even longer – on average four times longer than a women of normal weight.

Oestrogen is contained in fat cells, so the more fat cells you have the more oestrogen is present. When oestrogen levels are too high it can prevent ovulation and can also cause irregular and infrequent periods due to oestrogen interference. Similarly women who are underweight and who do not carry enough body fat cannot produce enough oestrogen to ovulate and menstruate. Elite female athletes with exceptionally low body fat will frequently encounter this problem. Inadequate nourishment puts a strain on a woman's body and can lower follicle stimulating hormone (FSH) and luteinising hormone (LH) levels. This leads to low levels of oestrogen and results in irregular menstrual cycles and follicles that are unable to develop properly and are inadequate for ovulation.

I frequently encounter clients at my clinic who are both overweight and undernourished. Although the client has a high intake of calories, when you take a closer look at his or her diet, it is lacking in nutrients. This double whammy can seriously interfere with fertility. In effect they may have all the problems related to being overweight and also many of the issues that usually relate to being underweight, because they are undernourished. If you stick to the guidelines of the Fertility Code Nutrition Plan this cannot happen and it is also inevitable that you will gravitate towards your ideal body weight, whilst enjoying all the benefits of a nutrient-rich diet.

For couples seeking assisted fertility treatments, evidence exists that being overweight has a negative impact on the outcome of their treatment. Women who are overweight do not generally respond as well to fertility medication and also have less success with IVF and other assisted reproductive technologies (ART) approaches. When the treatment is successful there is a higher rate of miscarriage for women who are overweight.

How can you stay motivated to achieve your ideal weight?

As much as you may want to improve your appearance and have all the benefits associated with a healthy body weight, the simple fact that once you address this issue you are far more likely to achieve a healthy pregnancy should provide enough motivation to stay on track with this nutrition plan. It is estimated that a staggering 75 per cent of women struggling with fertility caused by being overweight will conceive naturally once their weight has stabilised at normal levels (Silva et al, 1999). For women who are underweight and malnourished the figures are even more impressive, with 90 per cent of these women conceiving soon after they attain a normal body weight.

If you are overweight you should aim to lose about 1 to 2 lbs a week. This will help to ensure that you're losing fat. Losing more than a couple of pounds a week can indicate that you are losing fluid and burning muscle mass rather than fat. If you are aiming to lose weight you might be tempted to exercise strenuously in order to burn more calories. However, as we shall discuss later on, this is not conducive to increased fertility. When trying to reach your ideal body weight, the emphasis should be on eating the right foods.

Secrets to staying on track with the Nutrition Plan

- ♪ Eat breakfast every day
- ♪ Don't skip meals. Eat plenty of the allowed foods to keep hunger at bay
- ♪ Snack on seeds and dried apricots
- ♪ Stress can lead to comfort eating, so use the Fertility Code Mind Programme to destress
- ♪ Drink plenty of water
- ♪ Get lots of sleep. If you are tired during the day, you may crave sugar and other refined carbohydrates to give you an energy boost

♀♂

THE FERTILITY CODE NUTRITION PLAN EXPLAINED

Organic fruit and vegetables

Aim to eat ten portions of healthy organic fruit and vegetables every day

It is beyond doubt that fruit and vegetables are very good for you. They are crammed full of nutrients and you should aim to eat ten portions of fruit and vegetables every single day. Forget this silly five-a-day mantra – five is not enough. When you increase your intake to ten portions a day, you will provide your body with more of the healthy fibre, vitamins, minerals, antioxidants and phytonutrients necessary to stay healthy and conceive.

You should pay particular attention to including in your diet dark, leafy green vegetables such as spinach, cabbage, kale, rocket and broccoli. These greens contain beta-carotene, other B vitamins, vitamin E, iron, magnesium, zinc and selenium. They also contain the phytonutrient diindolylmethane (DIM), which has been proven to help both men and women to metabolise oestrogen. These vegetables can combat the oestrogen dominance that often leads to conditions such as polycystic ovary syndrome (PCOS) and endometriosis. For men, these foods help to regulate the testosterone/oestrogen balance and can improve sperm production.

The antioxidant beta-carotene is the nutrient most recognised as being important for fertility. This nutrient is found in carrots and sweet potatoes as well as greens such as broccoli and spinach. It helps to regulate menstruation and is central to maintaining the healthy hormone balance that prevents early miscarriage. In men it also helps to improve sperm quality.

Chinese medicine frequently associates first trimester miscarriage with a medical pattern known as xue xu (blood deficiency). Blood can be deficient because of any of three reasons: blood loss and inherited factors are two, but the more typical cause is improper diet. The problem is not so much the bad food that you eat but rather the good food that you do not eat enough of. In Chinese medicine the kings of the blood tonifying foods are – you guessed it – dark, leafy green vegetables. Someone who is not blood deficient should eat a fist size portion of greens every day. If you are blood deficient this should be increased to two fist-sized portions. For many people this can be quite challenging to achieve, so later in this chapter I suggest some supplements you can take to address this.

I specifically suggest that you try to eat organic fruit and vegetables because when you choose organic you avoid some of the pesticides, synthetic additives and chemical agents that contaminate our food. Many agricultural chemicals used on crops contain hormones, and, together with the hormones given to farm animals, these can affect our own hormonal balance and therefore our fertility.

There is also evidence that the levels of nutrients in many foods have decreased due to modern farming methods, which deplete the soil of nutrients. If the soil is depleted of nutrients, so too are the crops that come from that soil. Organic foods are therefore more likely to provide sufficient good quality nourishment to you and in turn to a new life.

Good fats versus bad fats

Replace bad fats with good fats

There are different kinds of fat, some are essential and some are harmful. This can be quite confusing as food producers frequently try to portray their products as healthy even when they contain harmful fats. Putting it simply, bad fats can damage your health and consequently your fertility, while good fats are in fact essential to enhancing your fertility.

You need to make an informed choice when it comes to eating fats. Eating the wrong fats can disrupt ovulation, induce insulin resistance, increase the risk of endometriosis and interfere with hormonal balance. All this is in addition to being generally harmful to your health. On the other hand eating good fats can enhance fertility in women and increase sperm volume and quality in men. Your body needs essential fats to produce hormones, combat inflammation and assist ovulation.

Two fats are generally classified as bad. These are trans fats and saturated fats. There is damning evidence against both of these fats and particularly against trans fats. The Fertility Code Nutrition Plan recommends that you keep saturated fat intake low and eliminate intake of all trans fats.

Saturated fats

Saturated fats are found in some of the most common foods, such as butter, cream, cheese, chocolate and red meat. Saturated fat is known to stimulate oestrogen production, which can compromise fertility. However, The Nurses' Health Study seemed to indicate that moderate amounts of saturated fats increased fertility. That being said, the same researchers also concluded that saturated fat intake should be kept below 17 g a day.

Other studies, such as Dr Cramner's study published in the *American Journal of Epidemiology* in 1994, have indicated that high intake of saturated fat tended to have a negative impact, particularly on women over thirty-five who were trying to conceive.

Amongst men, Harvard Medical School researched the typical British and Irish diet and found that high intake of saturated fat within a group of ninety-one men reduced their fertility rates by almost half, whether they were overweight or not (Attaman, 2012). Out of the ninety-one men twenty-one had problems with sperm count.

There is also evidence from The Nurses' Health Study that low-fat dairy foods may not be helpful to fertility. Other research had found that women who consumed a lot of low-fat dairy products such as skimmed milk were found to be almost twice as likely to suffer from period-related fertility problems when compared with those who consumed full-fat alternatives (Chavarro et al, 2007). However this study almost assumes that you must consume dairy products and this simply isn't true. The real truth is that you are much better advised to get your fats from oily fish and other sources rather than from dairy products.

Trans fats

Hydrogenated trans fats are artificially created by taking liquid oil and pumping hydrogen atoms into it at high temperatures over a period of hours until the liquid becomes semi solid. This process prevents the oil from becoming rancid but destroys its nutritional value. It also enables the manufacturer to convert cheap low-quality oils into butter substitutes, allowing them to improve their profit margin.

Because trans fats do not occur naturally, our bodies are simply unable to digest and deal with them properly and consequently they can become poisonous to important cellular reactions. Trans fats should be completely eliminated from your diet because they can significantly increase insulin resistance and cause ovulation problems. They also have been shown to interfere with hormone production and balance. The Nurses' Health Study found that women who consume as little as 4 g of trans fats a day were 70 per cent less likely to get pregnant than women who did not consume any.

There is no safe level of trans fats in your diet. If you are eating only fresh, natural foods you don't have to worry about trans fats, because they only exist in commercial, manufactured foods. Be cautious of commercially baked goods such as crackers, cakes, sweets, margarines and frozen meals. If you see the words 'hydrogenated' or 'partially hydrogenated' on the label, simply put it right back on the shelf. Some parts of the world have now recognised the full dangers of trans fats and have actually made it illegal to sell them. Trans fats are banned in New York City because of their harmful and deadly effects. However, it is still legal in the UK and Ireland to make and supply children's sweets containing these deadly fats.

Good fats

Good fats help sugar and insulin metabolism and therefore contribute to balancing hormones and supporting fertility. Essential fatty acids (EFAs) are, as the name suggests, essential to human health. EFAs are a vital component of every human cell, so they have many health benefits. In terms of fertility, they play an important role in supporting the follicle when it releases the egg and also in the production of sperm. Once pregnancy has been achieved they are also important for nourishing the growing embryo.

Essential fatty acids include:

- ⇲ **Omega-3** – found in oily fish, fish oils, dark leafy green vegetables, flaxseed and algae such as spirulina

- ⇲ **Omega-6** – found in vegetable oils, cereals, nuts and whole grains

- ⇲ **Omega-9** – found in olives, avocados and nuts (Omega-9 is technically not essential as our bodies can manufacture it if we have enough omega-3 and 6.)

Whilst essential omega-6's are inflammatory in their nature, omega-3's have anti-inflammatory qualities that are particularly supportive of fertility. The typical Western diet is rich in Omega 6's because they are so plentiful in oils and as a consequence we might even be getting too much of a good thing. Therefore we must place special emphasis on omega-3's as these EFAs in particular are helpful in supporting hormonal balance.

The message is clear: eating seafood is of considerable benefit in enhancing your fertility. The Fertility Code Nutrition Plan recommends that you eat at least three portions of oily fish every week, together with adequate portions of leafy green vegetables. If you dislike fish there are other options such as flaxseed, but in this case I would also recommend a good quality fish oil supplement.

Eat hormone-balancing food

Ensure phytoestrogens are part of your nutrition

Phytoestrogens are plant-based oestrogens that are believed to have a hormone-balancing effect. They are found in many of the foods supported elsewhere in this chapter and categorised as follows:

- ⇲ **Lignans** – found in nearly all vegetables and grains, one of the best sources being flaxseed

- ⇲ **Isoflavones** – found in legumes such as chickpeas, beans, lentils and soy

✤ **Coumestans** – found in alfalfa, pinto beans and mung beans

Phytoestrogens have been proven in studies throughout the world to lower cholesterol and prevent heart disease. They have also been shown to play a significant role in helping to maintain balanced male and female sex hormones.

There has been some evidence that consuming exceptionally large quantities of soya has a detrimental impact on fertility. However, consuming organic, as opposed to genetically modified, soya and limiting your intake to five portions a week has been shown to have a positive impact on fertility.

A recent study of IVF patients concluded that there were significant improvements in the number of pregnancies, the number of successful embryo implantations in the uterus, and the number of successful deliveries when women were given phytoestrogens to support their treatment (Unfer et al, 2004).

Implantation rates for those who were given phytoestrogens were about 25 per cent compared to 20 per cent confirmed pregnancy which compares favourably to just 21 per cent of those given progesterone alone. Nearly a third of those who had taken phytoestrogens had a successful pregnancy and a later delivery compared to just about 16 per cent of those who didn't receive phytoestrogens in the study.

Eat healthy sources of lean protein

Replace red and dark meat with healthier sources of protein

Protein plays an important role in your fertility by maintaining blood-sugar balance and providing the amino acids necessary for cellular repair. Protein also assists in the manufacture of hormones and in general provides for healthy reproductive function. You need a constant supply of protein, as it is not stored in your body. Therefore you should aim to eat nutrient-rich protein with every meal.

As our knowledge of nutrition and fertility has grown, we have become more aware that we should eat as low on the food chain as possible. Whilst many of us imagine that our ancestors hunted large wild beasts to survive, the truth is that we did not evolve eating large quantities of red meat. Throughout our evolution most of our diet came from plants, nuts, small game and fish. Although humans are omnivores, we lean far more towards being herbivores than carnivores. The great apes, our closest relatives in the animal kingdom, share approximately 97 per cent of our DNA and are 98 per cent vegetarian, and our own digestive system has evolved to cater for a predominantly vegetarian diet.

Excellent sources of protein include oily fish, eggs, pulses, beans and seeds. These high-quality foods should be our main sources of protein. Beans, nuts and seeds not only contain protein but are also rich in iron and fibre. The Nurses' Health Study revealed that women who got most of their protein from animal sources were 40 per cent more likely to encounter ovulation problems. By adding one serving of red meat, chicken or turkey a day to your diet you increase your risk of ovulation infertility by 30 per cent. It is disappointing that regular intake of white meats such as chicken and turkey also appear to have a detrimental impact on fertility. Recent studies have shown that the quality of these white meats has declined significantly in recent years, with the saturated fat content increasing by about 300 per cent over the last forty years. Unfortunately, organic poultry only shows a marginal improvement on these figures.

Studies have shown an increased risk of colon cancer in people who are heavy consumers of animal protein. The risk doubles when compared with those who consume smaller amounts of meat. But one wonders how this would compare to people who do not consume meat at all.

It has also been suggested that red meat consumption can increase susceptibility to fibroids and endometriosis. The saturated fats in red meat are inflammatory in nature, which can cause fertility problems. In one study on endometriosis it was shown that women who followed a diet high in animal protein were more likely to encounter problems conceiving and that when they did conceive they were less likely to carry the pregnancy to full term.

The Fertility Code Nutrition Plan recommendation is therefore to include fish, eggs, nuts, lentils and legumes as your protein staples. Avoid red meat completely and limit your intake of poultry to just two portions per week.

Avoid all dairy products

If it's not good enough for a cow it's not good enough for you

Cow's milk is really meant for calves, and babies are meant to drink their mother's milk until they are weaned from it. Nature has developed both types of milk and digestive systems accordingly. Humans are the only mammals that drink milk once they have reached adulthood, and even more strangely we drink the milk of a completely different species that is ten times our size. A calf, once it has matured, will no longer drink cow's milk. Humans, on the other hand, teach that after a mother has performed her nursing, a cow should take over. In other words humans are never weaned! This obviously doesn't make sense.

The enzymes used to break down and digest milk are lactase and renin. These enzymes are no longer present in most humans by the time they are three years old. There are also proteins in milk known as casein. There is considerably more casein found in cow's milk than in human milk. This tough, dense curd is difficult for humans to digest, and the goo hardens in the stomach and sticks to the lining of the intestines, preventing the absorption of nutrients. This can leave a large store of acidic, toxic mucus that lingers in the body, hampering digestion. A calf has four stomachs and nine feet of intestines. Our digestive system is simply not designed to break down cow's milk.

The sugar lactose, which is also found in milk, causes problems too. Many people are lactose intolerant and find it hard to digest. In fact less than 20 per cent of the world's population is believed to have the ability to digest lactose, by producing the enzyme lactase. If your body doesn't make lactase, and there is an 80 per cent chance it doesn't, then the milk sugar remains intact. Lactose cannot easily pass through the wall of the intestines into the bloodstream and so it remains in the intestines. Bacteria living in the gut jump on this energy source and feed on it. This can result in flatulence, bloating, stomach cramps and sometimes loose stools.

There have, however, been some studies that have indicated a beneficial effect of dairy products on fertility. It is likely that many participants in these studies had a background of nutrient deficiency, which was somehow improved by dairy consumption. Notwithstanding this, studies have also shown that the populations with the highest milk consumption also tend to be less fertile, particularly at older ages.

Another issue that should be considered is the possible effect of dairy products on hormones. Cows, like humans, produce milk only after giving birth. In order to keep dairy cows producing milk they are artificially inseminated. To keep the cow productive it is always either pregnant or has just given birth. This means that these cows have very high levels of oestrogen, some of which is passed on through its milk.

Drinking low-fat dairy is not a sensible alternative. A recent US study by Harvard Medical School found that women who consumed skimmed milk and low-fat dairy products were almost twice as likely to encounter fertility-related problems than those who consumed the full-fat alternatives.

As discussed in the previous section, it is very important to have fats in your diet, as they are necessary for the absorption of certain nutrients such as Vitamins A and E. However, the best sources of these essential fats are oily fish, nuts and seeds.

Avoid refined carbohydrates

Eat good slow carbs and ditch bad refined carbs

Refined carbohydrates are everywhere and the chief culprits are sugar, white bread and pasta, together with all the products made from these sources. You will find refined carbs in baked food (muffins, doughnuts, pastries, biscuits and cakes), white flour products (white bread and bagels), snack foods (sweets, crisps, pretzels), sweetened dairy products (ice cream, chocolate), soft drinks and concentrated fruit juices, and processed grain products, including many breakfast cereals.

Refined carbohydrates are generally considered bad news. They have little nutritional value and are in fact detrimental both to your general health and to fertility. Most processed foods will contain refined carbohydrates. These carbohydrates wreak havoc on your digestion and put your blood sugar on a roller coaster of highs and lows.

A particularly nasty variety of refined carbohydrate is high-fructose corn syrup. This is found in a wide variety of foods such as ketchup, juices and breakfast cereals. One of the most common causes of infertility in women is polycystic ovary syndrome (PCOS). PCOS often produces fluid-filled cysts on the outside of the ovaries and can shut down ovarian function. Many women with PCOS have insulin resistance, which is a breakdown in the cells' ability to respond to insulin. This can result in high levels of blood sugar and insulin, which causes many of the hormonal disturbances associated with the condition.

Insulin resistance and high blood sugar also carry implications even if you are not diagnosed with PCOS. A 1999 Danish study showed that the combination of high blood sugar and insulin resistance can significantly impair fertility in otherwise healthy women. This study showed that women with higher than average blood sugar levels were only half as likely to get pregnant as women with normal levels.

The Fertility Code Nutrition Plan substitutes whole grains and fruit and vegetables for refined carbohydrates. Whole grains are higher in beneficial fibre and vitamins, and fruit and vegetables provide other useful phytonutrients. This means that they are not only more nutritious in general, but they also help to control and sustain normal energy levels and appetite more effectively.

When you eliminate refined carbohydrates, you may experience some cravings as your body adjusts from the high-blood-sugar roller coaster. However, the more you reduce your intake of these foods the less you will crave them. You will no longer have those ups and downs in energy levels that are created by these foods.

Sugar: the worst carbohydrate for fertility

The average person in the UK and Ireland now consumes up to fifteen times the amount of sugar that would have been consumed one hundred years ago. This amounts to approximately thirty teaspoons of sugar per day. Most people don't have any idea that they are consuming so much, as it is hidden in a wide variety of processed foods. When you look more closely at what sugar is actually doing to your body you will think twice about how much you consume.

BAD CARBS	v	GOOD CARBS
White bread		Wholegrain bread
Regular pasta		Wholewheat pasta
White rice		Brown rice
Concentrated fruit juice		Fruit
Breakfast cereals		Oatmeal

Sugar and hormone disruption

Sugar causes sharp peaks and troughs in blood-sugar levels, which in turn leads to hormone imbalance and, potentially, fertility problems. A typical sugar roller-coaster day goes something like this: you eat a bar of chocolate, perhaps in the morning, and your body rapidly digests the sugar, giving an immediate energy rush. This feels pretty good for about fifteen to thirty minutes, but each time you do it your pancreas goes into overdrive and produces large amounts of insulin so that the sugar can be pushed out of your bloodstream and into your cells, where it is converted into energy. After this your blood-sugar levels collapse and you feel exhausted and deflated. At this point you might well crave more sugar, as you are drawn to try to achieve the same energy hit. Your adrenal glands will often compensate by releasing cortisol and adrenaline in order to help replenish your blood sugar. Cortisol is the stress hormone and this creates a fight or flight reaction in your body, which over time weakens your adrenal to the point where other endocrine glands are not signaled to release their hormones and the entire communication of the endocrine system becomes broken. You may produce lower levels of sex hormones. The repeated adrenal stimulation affects the levels of progesterone, oestrogen, testosterone and the androgen DHEA. This affects both men and women in equal measure. If you stay on this roller coaster for a long time you may develop insulin resistance.

Insulin resistance

Over-consumption of sugar causes the pancreas to release more and more insulin. Consistently releasing too much insulin is likely to ultimately cause insulin resistance. Insulin resistance may disrupt normal ovulation or limit the maturation process of the egg. It may also hinder the ability of the egg to implant in the uterus after conception. Women with insulin resistance are four to five times more likely to miscarry.

Yeast infection

Yeast infections may not directly cause fertility problems, but they can hinder the ability of the sperm to reach the egg. We do know that a diet that is high in sugar, or that includes large quantities of refined carbohydrates like white bread and pasta, can contribute to chronic yeast infections. A vaginal yeast infection can also make it almost impossible to have sexual intercourse.

Lowered immunity

Research has suggested that consuming just one tablespoon of sugar can lower your immunity for up to four hours at a time. Lowered immunity makes us more susceptible to infections of all kinds, including yeast infections and sexually transmitted diseases, all of which can significantly affect our fertility.

Vitamin and mineral depletion

For the body to continually release insulin, cortisol uses up vitamin and mineral stores, specifically the B vitamins (especially B6),

Vitamin E, magnesium and copper. Cortisol also interferes with the absorption of calcium and magnesium, which are important for fertility.

AVOID ADDITIVES, PRESERVATIVES AND CHEMICALS SUCH AS ARTIFICIAL SWEETENERS

Artificial sweeteners and additives: deadly chemicals

Aspartame (E951) is a widely used artificial sweetener that has been linked to fertility problems and birth defects. In general steer clear of all artificial sweeteners as they make your body too acidic and have been linked to a wide variety of health problems.

The Food and Drugs Administration (FDA) in the United States took sixteen years to approve aspartame because of concerns about its safety for human consumption. It has been linked to a wide variety of symptoms, including headaches, panic attacks, depression, seizures, multiple sclerosis and cancer. Aspartame is made from wood alcohol, and another artificial sweetener, saccharin, is made from petroleum. These are widely used in diet drinks and low-calorie processed foods. These processed foods are usually promoted as healthy choices and you will see these ingredients in many low-fat, low-calorie yoghurts and desserts. Studies have shown that women who consume these forms of low-calorie products have significantly increased incidence of infertility (Chavarro et al, 2007).

One reason why someone would consume these sweeteners is that they are trying to control their weight for fertility reasons. However, a side effect of these sweeteners is that they elicit carbohydrate cravings, so often the net result of using artificial sweeteners is a tendency to gain weight.

All in all, there is no good reason to include artificial sweeteners in your diet and every reason to avoid them. An acceptable alternative to sugar is a moderate amount of organic honey and the natural sweetness you obtain from fruit.

DRINK PLENTY OF WATER AND RESTRICT ALCOHOL CONSUMPTION

Don't wait until you are thirsty to drink water

Water plays a major role in the production of energy and whilst we can survive without food for weeks, we can only survive for a few days without water. By the time you are thirsty you are already dehydrated. The human body is 60 per cent water and a regular intake is crucial to maintaining a healthy hormonal balance. Water also supports kidney function. If you are drinking enough water, your urine should be pretty clear and colourless. This is a good sign, as if your urine is dark it frequently means that you have allowed yourself to become somewhat dehydrated.

So first of all never allow yourself to get thirsty, and drink regularly throughout the day. You should aim to drink around two litres of water every day. If you are exercising you should drink more. Do try to stop drinking about three hours before you go to bed, however. This will give your body time to empty your bladder before you fall asleep. Sleep is also important, so I don't want you getting up in the middle of the night to go to the bathroom.

Where you should you get your water from is the next thing to consider. Despite all assurances I don't believe that unfiltered tap water is a good source, as it frequently contains residues of harmful chemicals that can wreak havoc with your hormonal balance. These chemicals include benzene, pesticides and disinfectant by-products. Chemicals seep into our water supplies from waste-disposal sites, as well as from pesticides that are swept into lakes and streams from nearby land. However, I do not recommend bottled mineral water either, as it frequently contains such high levels of radioactivity, nitrates and other pollutants that it would be illegal if it came out of a tap.

My preferred approach is to filter tap water through a standard charcoal filter, which will remove most of the harmful substances at a very low cost. You could also invest in a point-of-use filter, which you can fit to your kitchen sink. This will treat all the water you use in your kitchen and is the optimal way of filtering your water, although it is a little more expensive.

You shouldn't drink water that is too cold. Chinese medicine understands that cold water can strain your digestive system as your body works to heat it up.

What about soft drinks? Well, most soft drinks contain high levels of refined carbohydrate or artificial sweeteners, which we know have a hugely detrimental effect on our bodies. Apart from this, soft drinks do not provide the same level of hydration as water. As soft drinks contain significant amounts of sugar, artificial sweeteners and phosphates, they also have a dehydrating effect on the body.

Alcohol

An occasional glass of wine (i.e. one or two a week) probably won't hurt your odds of conceiving. Research has shown that when this rises above five glasses a week it can interfere with ovulation and menstruation, making it more difficult to conceive. One large study concluded that limiting alcohol intake to fewer than five units a week meant you were twice as likely to get pregnant in a six month period as someone who drank more than this (Jensen et al, 1998). A similar study concluded that men who regularly drank alcohol also took twice as long to successfully conceive when compared to men who didn't drink at all. We know that alcohol can damage sperm quality, lower sperm motility and increase abnormalities. Alcohol also reduces sperm count and can lower testosterone levels. Most studies have therefore concluded that the more alcohol consumed, the greater the decrease in fertility.

For couples electing to use assisted reproductive technologies such as IVF, I recommended not drinking any alcohol for one month prior to IVF, and of course continuing to abstain after the transfer has taken place. If you continue to drink at this time you significantly increase your risk of the treatment failing, and if you are successful it more than doubles the risk of miscarriage. This generally applies to both the man and the woman.

Alcohol also interferes with your body's ability to absorb nutrients and at a time when you are trying to do everything possible to be healthy, it makes no sense to spoil your efforts by drinking large amounts of alcohol. Alcohol has been shown to interfere with the absorption of zinc, which is critical for male fertility, and the absorption of folic acid, which plays a crucial role in bringing the egg to maturity for ovulation. In addition, alcohol generally acidifies the body and it is believed that if cervical mucus becomes too acidic, this can prevent the sperm surviving long enough to reach the egg.

All in all I would support the approach of avoiding alcohol completely if you are trying to get pregnant and especially if you achieve pregnancy. If, however, you limit your intake to no more than two glasses of wine per week you are probably going to be fine.

Replace coffee and tea with green or jasmine tea

It is established that the caffeine found in coffee can reduce the flow of blood to the uterus, which can also interfere with implantation. Drinking coffee also increases the risk of clotting and, consequently, miscarriage. As caffeine is a stimulant, coffee also has a tendency to increase stress and anxiety and it can hamper your ability to sleep well at night.

The research on whether coffee affects fertility is mixed, but experts generally agree that low coffee consumption (one mug a day) won't get in the way of getting pregnant. If, however, you are undergoing IVF I would be inclined to avoid coffee completely as the effect of caffeine on the blood vessels (slowing blood flow to the uterus) can potentially make it harder for the egg to grab hold. One Dutch study established that drinking four cups of coffee a day lowered a woman's chances of having a baby by 25 per cent. This is equivalent to the reduction in fertility caused by smoking heavily and being very overweight.

I recommend that you switch from coffee to green or jasmine tea when you are trying to get pregnant. One of the primary benefits of green tea with regard to fertility is not in what it contains, but rather in what it does not contain. Green tea contains much less caffeine than regular tea or coffee. Two of the main ingredients in green tea, hypoxanthine and polyphenols, may actually lead to a higher percentage of viable embryos, according to recent research. Other research has suggested that these compounds help with the maturing of eggs, and may even make eggs more fertile. Polyphenols also serve as antioxidants, which help protect your body from a variety of conditions.

Replace refined table salt with healthier spices

Salt is necessary for the proper functioning of the body. It helps maintain the fluid in your blood cells and it is used to transmit signals through our nerves and muscles. It is also used in the absorption of certain nutrients from the small intestine. Our bodies cannot make salt, so we rely on food as a source. However, just 500 mg of dietary sodium supplies our body's daily needs. On average we consume fifteen times the required daily amount of dietary sodium we need. This can lead to hypertension and cause mineral deficiencies with regard to calcium, magnesium and potassium. Too much salt can also hamper your fertility. Tests carried out on animals showed that when they were fed a diet high in salt it impaired ovulation, increased blood pressure and reduced fertility.

In addition to the salt we add to our food, many foods contain sodium as part of their normal chemical composition. Ingredients such as baking powder, baking soda, soy sauce, pickles and olives contain significant amounts of sodium. The chemical additives contained in processed foods can contain exceptionally large amounts of sodium – monosodium glutamate, sodium phosphate, sodium nitrate and sodium benzoate, to name but a few.

With the Fertility Code Nutrition Plan you will stop using table salt. As you will also be avoiding processed foods, you will simply get adequate sodium from natural sources. If you still wish to season food to add taste, you should add the following healthy alternatives: basil, bay leaves, cayenne, cinnamon, dill seeds, garlic, ginger, mustard seeds, paprika, parsley, pepper, saffron, thyme and turmeric.

♀ ♂

FOOD TABLE

	Good Choice	Avoid	Limit Intake
Alfalfa	✓		
Apple	✓		
Apricots	✓		
Artichokes	✓		
Asparagus	✓		
Aubergine	✓		
Avocado	✓		
Bagel		✗	
Baked Beans		✗	
Banana	✓		
Barley	✓		
Bean Curd	✓		
Beef		✗	
Beetroot	✓		
Biscuits		✗	
Black Beans	✓		
Bok Choi	✓		
Broccoli	✓		
Brown Rice	✓		
Brussels Sprouts	✓		
Buckwheat	✓		
Butter Beans	✓		
Cabbage	✓		
Cakes		✗	
Carrots	✓		
Cashew Nuts	✓		
Cauliflower	✓		
Celery	✓		
Cereal Bars		✗	
Cheese		✗	
Cherries	✓		
Chicken, Organic Free Range			◇ Limit to 2 portions of poultry per week

	Good Choice	Avoid	Limit Intake
Chicken Nuggets		x	
Chickpeas	✓		
Chillies		x	
Chives	✓		
Chocolate		x	
Coffee		x	
Cola Drinks		x	
Commercial Breakfast Cereals		x	
Corn	✓		
Corn Flakes		x	
Courgette	✓		
Cranberries	✓		
Croissant		x	
Cucumber	✓		
Custard		x	
Dates	✓		
Diet Soft Drinks		x	
Digestive Biscuits		x	
Duck		x	
Eggs, Organic Free Range	✓		
Fennel	✓		
Fish (oily)	✓		
French Fries		x	
Fruit Juice (concentrated)		x	
Fruit Juice (fresh)	✓		
Garlic	✓		
Grapefruit	✓		
Grapes	✓		
Green Beans	✓		
Ham		x	
Hamburger		x	
Honey			◇ Moderate intake of organic honey is a good replacement for sugar
Hummus	✓		
Ice Cream		x	

	Good Choice	Avoid	Limit Intake
Jam		x	
Jelly		x	
Kale	✓		
Kidney Beans	✓		
Kiwi	✓		
Lamb		x	
Leeks	✓		
Lemon	✓		
Lentils	✓		
Lettuce	✓		
Lime	✓		
Mango	✓		
Marmalade		x	
Milk, Full Fat		x	
Milk, Semi Skimmed		x	
Milk, Skimmed		x	
Muffins		x	
Mung Beans	✓		
Mushrooms	✓		
Noodles	✓		
Oats	✓		
Onions	✓		
Orange	✓		
Orange Juice	✓		
Parsnips	✓		
Pasta, Organic Wholewheat only	✓		
Peach	✓		
Peanuts	✓		
Pear	✓		
Peppers	✓		
Pineapple	✓		
Pinto Beans	✓		
Pitta Bread, Wholemeal only	✓		
Pizza		x	
Plum	✓		

	Good Choice	Avoid	Limit Intake	
Popcorn		x		
Pork		x		
Porridge	✓			
Potatoes			◇	Raises insulin levels so eat in moderation
Pretzels		x		
Prunes	✓			
Pumpkin	✓			
Raisins	✓			
Rhubarb	✓			
Rice, Brown	✓			
Rocket	✓			
Rye Bread	✓			
Salami		x		
Salmon, Wild	✓			
Sardines	✓			
Sausages		x		
Scallops		x		Prone to toxic contamination
Sesame Seeds	✓			
Shallots	✓			
Shellfish		x		Prone to toxic contamination
Soft Drinks		x		
Soy Beans, Organic only			◇	Limit to 5 portions of soy based products per week
Soya Milk, Organic only			◇	Limit to 5 portions of soy based products per week
Spaghetti, Organic Wholewheat only	✓			
Spinach	✓			
Spring Onions	✓			
Steak		x		
Strawberries	✓			
Stuffing, Bread		x		
Sugar		x		
Sultanas	✓			

	Good Choice	Avoid	Limit Intake	
Sweet Potato	✓			
Tea, English			◇	
Tea, Green	✓			
Tea, Jasmine	✓			
Tofu, Organic only			◇	Limit to 5 portions of soy based products per week
Tomato	✓			
Trout	✓			
Tuna		✗		Avoid due to risk of toxins
Turkey, Organic			◇	Limit to 2 portions of poultry per week
Veal		✗		
Vinegar	✓			
Waffles		✗		
Watercress	✓			
Watermelon	✓			
White Bread		✗		
Wholemeal Bread	✓			
Yoghurt		✗		

♀ ♂

THE FERTILITY CODE SUPPLEMENTS

The first thing to say is that when it comes to nutrients it is best to focus your attention on getting these vital vitamins and minerals from the food you eat. The Fertility Code Nutrition Plan ensures that you will be getting a healthy supply of nutrients from the best source – healthy food.

So why use supplements? Farmed soils have become increasingly depleted in a number of vital nutrients, and as a result our plants, fruit and vegetables are often lacking in a variety of essential nutrients. Chemical fertilisers can cause toxic harm to our bodies but they are also effective at stimulating crop growth within these nutrient-poor soils. This results in the soils becoming increasingly depleted even though the crops continue to grow. Although the vegetables appear to flourish, they are frequently lacking in the full range of minerals and vitamins.

So, while the best way to get vitamins and minerals is through a high-quality, varied organic diet, when you want to optimise your fertility it also makes sense to support your diet with a basic programme of supplementation. This will ensure that you don't have any gaps in your diet and will also provide some additional benefits that might be difficult to achieve from diet alone.

The following supplement programme is part of the Fertility Code Nutrition Plan.

NUTRIENTS	FEMALE PARTNER	MALE PARTNER
Spirulina	6000 mg	6000 mg
Folic acid	400 mcg	800 mcg
Calcium	1000 mg	1000 mg
Zinc	30 mg	30 mg
Selenium	100 mcg	100 mcg
Omega-3 Fish Oil	1000 mg	1000 mg
Vitamin C	2000 mg	2000 mg
Vitamin D	5000 IU	5000 IU
Vitamin E	400 IU	400 IU
L-arginine	350 mg	500 mg

Spirulina

Taking spirulina, commonly referred to as blue-green algae, is an excellent way to support fertility and pregnancy because of its superior nutritional content. The protein in spirulina is considered to be of the highest quality, superior to all other plant proteins, including those in the legume family (beans, peas, soy, etc.). It is an excellent source of vitamins, minerals, amino acids, fatty acids, beta carotene, chlorophyll, and even various phytochemicals. It also stimulates the growth of good bacteria, like Bifidus.

Spirulina helps control hormones. It has been proven to be effective in correcting hormonal imbalances, which can help to increase fertility. This also helps you to control your weight, which helps conception, as obesity can be a cause of infertility.

Dosage: 6,000 mg per day for men and women

Folic acid

Folic acid is frequently used to prevent spina bifida in babies. We now know that this important supplement protects against a variety of neural tube defects (NTDs), which are malformations of the brain and central nervous system. Babies develop their neural tube, which later becomes the brain and spinal cord, during the first weeks of pregnancy and folic acid supports this. A pregnancy in which an NTD is present is highly likely to result in miscarriage and folic acid offers protection against this. Women should take 400 mg for at least two months before conception and at least until the twelfth week of pregnancy.

Folic acid also offers significant fertility benefits for men. A study published in the *Journal of Human Reproduction* found that men who consumed a higher than recommended daily amount of folic acid had a significantly lower frequency of abnormal sperm (Forges et al, 2007). Researchers in California established that men who consumed between 722 and 1,150 mcg had a 20 to 30 per cent reduction in abnormal sperm. I would therefore recommend that men should take 800 mcg of folic acid daily.

Not only does folic acid help to prevent neural tube defects in unborn babies it also reduces the risk of anaemia, heart disease, depression and Alzheimer's.

Dosage: 400 mcg per day for women

800 mcg per day for men

Calcium

Calcium is well known for helping to support strong bones and healthy teeth but it is also essential for getting pregnant.

Studies have established calcium's roll in conception (Taylor,

1994). It has been proven that calcium is a vital ingredient in the process of triggering growth in embryos. Calcium in the surrounding fluid helps the embryo to develop.

A second study focused on what triggers sperm to abruptly convert their swimming style from a slow and steady swim, using side-to-side motion, to the whip-cracking snap that thrusts them into the egg. Researchers found that when sperm arrived in the alkaline environment of the reproductive tract, it triggers the tails' whip-like motion. Calcium helps to create an alkaline environment in the reproductive tract. The sperm soaks up calcium, which causes it to thrust towards the egg.

Dosage: 1,000 mg per day for men and women

Zinc

Zinc is considered the most important mineral for fertility in both men and women. It is the most widely studied nutrient in terms of fertility and is an essential component of genetic material. Zinc deficiency can cause chromosome changes in both partners, leading to reduced fertility and an increased risk of miscarriage.

For women zinc is necessary for your body to use effectively the reproductive hormones, oestrogen and progesterone.

For men, zinc is found in high concentrations in the sperm. Zinc is needed to make the outer layer and tail of the sperm and is therefore essential for the health of sperm and, subsequently, your baby. Several studies have shown that increasing zinc in a man's diet will frequently increase his sperm count.

Dosage: 30 mg per day for men and women

Selenium

Selenium plays a critical role in the production of antioxidant enzymes that protect cells against the effects of free radicals produced during normal oxygen metabolism. It also protects your body against the harmful effects of free radicals generated by smoke, pollution, radiation and other environmental toxins. Selenium is therefore essential for normal functioning of the immune system and can also prevent chromosome breakage, which is known to be a cause of birth defects and miscarriages. In addition to all this, selenium is involved in iodine metabolism, pancreatic function and DNA repair.

Dosage: 100 mcg per day for both men and women

Omega-3 fish oils

We have already spoken about essential fatty acids and their importance in your diet. I believe there is merit in taking an omega-3 EFA supplement to support your normal nutritional intake. These essential fats have a profound effect on every system of the body, including the reproductive system, and they are crucial for healthy hormone function.

Omega-3 fats help to regulate the reproductive hormones. Recent studies have established that the consumption of fish oil significantly improves fertility in both men and women (Saldeen, 2004). Fish oil is typically harvested from cold-water fish like salmon, trout, sardines and a wide variety of others. These oils contain high concentrations of omega-3 fatty acids, which play a key role in the motility of sperm. Sperm cells face a long and arduous journey before they even attempt to penetrate an ovum. In order to have the best chance of success, they must be, first of all, plentiful, and, second of all, up to the task. The more sperm that make it to the ovum (millions will die naturally during the journey), the better chance there will be that one of them will successfully fertilise the egg. Consumption of omega-3 fish oils also increases blood flow to the genitals, which leads to an increase in the production of sperm, as well as a decrease in the likelihood of erectile dysfunction.

For women there are certain conditions that the body can bring about that help her to become more fertile. The consumption of fish oil promotes the natural occurrence of these conditions. For example, one of the main components of fertility is a regular and predictable menstrual cycle. Consumption of fish oils helps to promote a regular menstrual cycle. Fish oils also enhance the body's natural reactions during the menstrual cycle. A woman's body temperature, for example, naturally increases during ovulation. This is a major tell-tale signal that her body is ready to conceive. By encouraging this natural surge in temperature, fish oil can increase the chances of successfully conceiving.

Dosage: 1,000 mg per day for both men and women

Vitamin C

Vitamin C is one of the most potent antioxidants known to science and is a powerful free-radical scavenger. Studies have shown that vitamin C enhances sperm quality, protecting sperm and the DNA within it from damage. Some research has indicated that certain types of DNA damage in the sperm can make it difficult to conceive in the first place, or increase the risk of miscarriage if conception does take place. If DNA is damaged, there may be a chromosomal problem, should pregnancy occur. Whether or not DNA damage has these effects has not been conclusively proven, but it's worth taking vitamin C and the other antioxidants as a precautionary measure.

Vitamin C also appears to prevent sperm from clumping together, making them more motile.

Dosage: 2,000 mg per day for both men and women

Vitamin D

Whilst most people associate vitamin D with bone health, a number of studies have shown that vitamin D has a direct impact on both male and female fertility. In men, vitamin D helps in the production of testosterone, the hormone chiefly responsible for the production of sperm. In women, vitamin D works directly on the ovaries, helping to regulate how oestrogen is used to help egg follicles develop.

Vitamin D also appears to play a role in how oestrogen acts in the uterus, particularly with regard to the development of the lining. When vitamin D levels are low the uterus lining may not be sufficiently thick to hold on to the embryo. This can ultimately lead to miscarriage.

Vitamin D is now considered such an important nutrient in fertility that Yale University devoted an entire study to learning what happens when levels decline. They studied sixty-seven women who had problems conceiving and found that 93 per cent of them had low levels of vitamin D. According to researcher Dr Lubna Pal, 'Not a single patient with either ovulatory disturbance or polycystic ovary syndrome demonstrated normal vitamin D levels; 39 per cent of those with ovulatory disturbance and 38 per cent of those with PCOS had levels consistent with deficiency.'

In another study women who lost their menstrual cycle and were considered infertile due to PCOS resumed their periods and became pregnant when vitamin D levels were increased.

Vitamin D is also crucial to controlling blood levels of calcium. When calcium levels go down, the rate of pre-menstrual syndrome (PMS) goes up. More importantly, however, the reverse is also true – when calcium levels are sufficient, PMS is reduced, which means fertility generally improves.

So what's the connection between PMS and fertility? When PMS is under control you will simply feel better and less stressed, which in turn means that all hormone activity will be better balanced. But more importantly, as PMS is a condition that is underscored by hormone imbalance, dealing with this problem helps ensure the proper hormone balance necessary for pregnancy.

Finally, very recent research shows that vitamin D deficiencies may be linked to a higher rate of bacterial vaginosis (BV), a very common infection that has been linked to infertility. Indeed, not only can this infection create a hostile environment that can negatively impact sperm, if left untreated BV can quickly turn into the more serious condition pelvic inflammatory disease (PID). This infection can easily spread into the fallopian tubes, ovaries and even the uterus, and not only directly and immediately have an impact on your ability to get pregnant, but also create scar tissue that continues to interfere with conception long after the infection clears. As well as this, if you become pregnant while you have a BV infection, it could increase your risk of miscarriage and lead to premature labour and a low birth-weight baby.

Dosage: 5,000 IU per day for both men and women

Vitamin E

Vitamin E is a powerful antioxidant and it also plays a role in conception. We've spoken about antioxidants a few times now, but what are they? Antioxidants counteract the damaging effects of oxidation. Oxidation takes place when oxygen reacts with other molecules in the body. Just like oxygen reacts with metal to cause rust. Free radicals are by-products of reactions in the body, and can cause damage, which accumulates over time. Antioxidants neutralise free radicals and prevent them from causing damage.

Our reproductive cells are very susceptible to oxidative damage. Sperm cells are particularly susceptible to damage, however this can be rectified relatively quickly, as sperm is continually replenished. It is believed that the antioxidant element of vitamin E might help to improve sperm quality.

Women's reproductive cells also benefit from vitamin E. Whilst women are born with all the eggs they will ever have, they lie dormant until recruited for development. So although these eggs are as old as the woman, they really haven't been active all that time. However, during the process of maturation, they can be damaged by free radicals. Taking an antioxidant like vitamin E can help prevent this damage.

Couples undergoing IVF treatment have shown increased fertilisation rates when they supplement with vitamin E.

Dosage: 400 IU per day for both men and women

L-arginine

L-arginine is an essential amino acid that helps to support healthy blood circulation. It has also been shown to offer fertility benefits in both men and women. Studies have established that supplementing with L-arginine can bring about the following:

- ✎ Improved blood flow to the uterus and ovaries
- ✎ Improved production of cervical mucus
- ✎ Enhanced libido
- ✎ Increased testosterone levels in men

This is an amino acid found in many foods. The head of the sperm contains a large amount of this nutrient, which is essential for sperm production. Supplementing with L-arginine may help increase both sperm count and quality.

Dosage: 350 mg per day for women

500 mg per day for men

Note: People who have herpes attacks (either cold sores or genital herpes) should not supplement with L-arginine because it stimulates the virus.

HOW TO PREPARE AND EAT YOUR FOOD

As well as eating the correct foods, the Fertility Code places emphasis on preparing and eating food in the healthiest manner. The following is a step-by-step approach to buying, preparing and eating food in a way that will help you to get the maximum benefit from it.

- Variety is encouraged as much as possible. This makes it easier to follow the plan because your diet will be varied and interesting.

- There should be a preference for fresh ingredients. Fresh organic vegetables are preferred over frozen vegetables.

- Always wash your fruit and vegetables thoroughly to help remove chemical pesticides.

- Ingredients should be diced, shredded and thinly sliced, as this helps digestion.

- The best methods of cooking are stir-frying and steaming. These methods cook faster and preserve more nutrients.

- Foods should be served at or above room temperature, and you should avoid eating direct from the fridge, as Chinese medicine sees cold food as hampering digestion.

✤ Meals can be followed with a warm cup of green or jasmine tea, as these are considered an aid to digestion. Warm water is also good for this purpose.

✤ You should avoid overeating, as this puts strain on your digestion. Eat only to the point that you are 80 per cent full. Eat little and often and choose quality over quantity.

✤ Breakfast is the most important meal of the day and you should aim to stop eating before 6 p.m. This is easier to do if you are going to bed at a reasonable time also. By eating larger meals earlier in the day your body has a greater chance to burn off these calories. More importantly, by not eating a heavy meal close to bedtime your body is able to rest and recover better as resources are not being used to digest your food.

✤ Sit down and try to relax when you are eating. Try to avoid eating on the run and working lunches, as these activities impair digestion.

♀♂

CHAPTER SUMMARY

Making the correct food choices is one of the most powerful things you can do to enhance your health and your fertility. It is the key to attaining optimum nutrition for fertility. Some people try to adjust their diets very slowly, but if your diet contains a lot of poor food choices, with lots of fast food and processed food, I think it is much easier to make one big adjustment than to make smaller changes. A big adjustment that delivers benefits more quickly provides more encouragement and better motivation. You will feel better much more quickly.

Be aware that the food industry constantly tries to fool you into thinking some foods are good even when they are not. Choose good fats over bad fats, healthier complex carbohydrates over refined carbohydrates and avoid dairy, salt and too much alcohol.

Although supplements should never replace healthy nutrition, there is still merit in taking certain vitamin and mineral supplements to support your nutrition.

There are many delicious menu options open to you when putting into practice the Fertility Code Nutrition Plan. For a free detailed list of these menu options and recipes please register online on our website www.fertilitycode.com

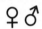

THE
Fertility CODE
Detox

"The best way to detoxify is to stop putting toxic things into the body and depend upon its own mechanisms"

Andrew Weil M.D.

INTRODUCTION

Toxins are everywhere. They are in the food we eat, the water we drink, the air we breathe, the lotions and sprays we put on our skin. We are not merely inhabitants of a toxic world; we can also be active participants depending on how we choose to live our lives.

However, we are not defenceless in this toxic world. Despite all the toxicity that surrounds us, plants still grow, flowers still bloom, animals still thrive and people still have families. Finding a way to eliminate toxins from your body is one of the most effective ways to rejuvenate your health, and in doing so, increase your fertility.

Our bodies can be contaminated by a variety of sources: pollution in our water supply, the air we breathe, the food we eat, the clothes we wear, the houses we live in. We are exposed to toxins every day of our lives. Our bodies must contend with thousands of pollutants and chemicals that we come into contact with all the time. But our bodies are designed to deal with these toxins: it's just that sometimes the cumulative effect – or toxic load – becomes too much. When this happens our bodies finally start to break down and problems occur. Toxic overload can occur at any time and symptoms can include asthma, allergies, lowered immunity, skin problems, fatigue, as well as a host of other conditions.

Decreasing your toxic exposure and toxic load takes time and awareness, not to mention commitment. In this chapter we will examine ways in which you can achieve this. Depending on your exposure to toxic elements, this part of the Fertility Code will vary from person to person. Whatever your personal toxic load, though, by making changes to unhelpful habits and behavioural patterns, in a relatively short space of time you can dramatically improve your health and enhance your fertility.

Case study – Susan and Paul

Susan was thirty-five when she came to my clinic. She and her husband, Paul, had been trying to conceive for almost four years and were soon to commence a second course of IVF. She wanted to become as healthy as possible prior to embarking on this next stage of her journey.

During the initial consultation it was apparent that there were many aspects of Susan's lifestyle that could be hampering her chances of successfully conceiving. Susan's eating habits were very poor and she smoked twenty cigarettes a day. She rarely ate breakfast and she got through each morning on a supply of coffee, chocolate and nicotine. When the afternoon slump hit, she would again turn to coffee and sugar. In fact, each day she drank an average of seven mugs of coffee.

Even though she skipped meals, her tendency to eat lots of sugary foods and refined carbohydrates meant that she was at least 20 lbs overweight. Tired after a day's work, when they got home in the evening Susan and Paul would often turn to what she called the 'easy option' and either eat a take-away or some ready-made processed meal.

Not surprisingly Susan had a whole host of symptoms that reflected her lifestyle. These included poor immunity, digestive problems, fatigue, skin problems and poor sleep patterns.

Susan and Paul were absolutely determined to do whatever they could to optimise their chances and they agreed to a complete overhaul of their lifestyle. This involved changing behaviours, eliminating toxins such as coffee and nicotine and dramatically improving their diet.

Within four weeks all of Susan's symptoms had virtually disappeared and she felt completely revitalised. Within three months she was back to her optimum weight for the first time in years and felt ready to embark on her IVF journey, knowing that she was in a much better place than when she first visited the clinic. Susan's IVF treatment was successful and just a year after she visited the clinic they had a healthy baby boy.

EVERYDAY TOXINS

Some toxins are highly poisonous chemicals and are dangerous in even small amounts. Most of the toxins we will deal with in the Fertility Code Detox are only damaging when our body's ability to metabolise and excrete these substances is overwhelmed.

Environmental toxins

Environmental toxins come from external sources. These toxins are absorbed through the food we eat, the fluids we drink, the air we breathe and whatever we put on our skin. The toxins in our food enter our bodies through the digestive system and move on to the liver, where they are filtered and prepared for excretion. Some examples of environmental toxins potentially harmful to our fertility include:

Hormones in food – The food we eat is a source of a variety of nutrients, chemicals, hormones and hormone-like substances. Hormones in meat, dairy and endocrine disrupting pesticides can mimic the activity of your own endocrine hormones and disrupt normal function.

Endocrine disruptors – Endocrine disruptors are substances that interfere with our body's hormonal or endocrine system and cause damage to our neurological, immune and reproductive functions. These toxins are therefore associated with fertility issues and with other serious health issues. They can be found in many substances such as pesticides, plastics, industrial by-products and environmental pollution.

Whilst food toxins must be ingested, usually in large amounts, before they cause problems, these pollutants can act even in small concentrations in our body. Many scientists now believe that small amounts of endocrine disruptors have the potential to cause enormous damage. Common endocrine-disrupting chemicals are not widely recognised by their names but we would do well to understand and avoid them to enhance fertility.

Metabolic toxins

You may not realise it, but we are our own main source of toxicity.

The by-products of normal cell metabolism and other physiological processes are all toxic when they are not processed properly. Improper diet, excess body weight, stress and poor digestion can all allow these toxins to build up and cause disease. Some examples of toxins that result from our own metabolic processes include the production of excessive amounts of hormones such as insulin and oestrogen, and the by-products of chronic inflammation.

Too much oestrogen in a woman's body is believed to be a contributing factor towards infertility, endometriosis and fibroids. During childbearing years oestrogen is produced in the ovaries and the fat cells. Body fat is biologically active, which means that when a woman is overweight she may produce excessively high levels of oestrogen.

Another hormone, insulin, is released by the pancreas in response to eating a meal and readies our cells to transport newly available blood sugar into the cells. If you eat too many refined carbohydrates over extended periods, insulin levels climb and the cells lose their ability to respond to the metabolic message. This can lead to a condition called insulin resistance, which threatens fertility.

Insulin is important for digestion and for immediate energy needs. It sends excess glucose to the liver, the muscles and to the red blood cells, where it is stored as glycogen for use later on. The uterus also stores glycogen during pregnancy, which is used to nourish the embryo. When glycogen stores are full, the liver takes the glycogen and turns it into a triglyceride, or a fat cell, and it is then stored as fat tissue. Sustained excessive production of insulin can lead ultimately to developing diabetes and a whole host of medical problems associated with this condition, such as frequent urination, excessive thirst, increased fatigue, frequent infections and poor healing. Insulin is understood to be chemically similar to the reproductive hormones, which is believed to cause confusion to the endocrine system. This can disrupt the reproductive system and is believed to contribute to infertility in both men and women.

Stress toxins – The stress hormone cortisol is secreted by the adrenal glands and has evolved as the human response to danger. Small increases of cortisol can be beneficial as they:

 ✎ provide a sudden burst of energy for survival reasons

- ♮ improve memory and concentration
- ♮ increase immunity
- ♮ elevate the pain threshold
- ♮ help maintain homeostasis in the body

While cortisol is an important and helpful part of the body's response to stress, it's important that our relaxation response is also activated so the body's functions can return to normal following a stressful event. However, due to the pressures of modern living, our high-stress culture and constant contact with work via mobile phone and internet, our stress response is activated so often that the body doesn't always have a chance to return to normal, resulting in a state of chronic stress.

When higher levels of cortisol are in the bloodstream over a longer period of time (like those associated with chronic stress) it can have negative effects such as:

- ♮ impaired cognitive performance
- ♮ suppressed thyroid function
- ♮ blood-sugar imbalances such as hyperglycemia
- ♮ decreased bone density
- ♮ decreased muscle tissue
- ♮ high blood pressure
- ♮ lowered immunity, inflammatory responses and slow wound healing
- ♮ increased abdominal fat

THE GOOD NEWS: YOU CAN AVOID TOXINS AND REMOVE THEM FROM YOUR BODY

We can take steps to minimise our exposure to toxic elements. The Fertility Code Detox provides an effective strategy for enhancing your body's ability to manage and remove environmental and internal toxins.

Our body manages toxins in several ways. The lymphatic, circulatory and respiratory systems, together with the skin and sweat glands, mechanically manage and process toxins in our body.

The lymphatic system

The lymphatic system is directly involved in your immune response. It is your body's waste management system, collecting excess fluid, debris, used blood cells, pathogens and other toxins from the fluid that surrounds the cells within your body. This fluid is known as interstitial fluid and it contains the by-products of cellular metabolism, hormone metabolites and components of the immune system. Once the debris is collected in the lymph vessels, the fluid is called lymph and it circulates below the skin. The lymph then passes through special processing structures called lymph nodes and enters the blood.

The lymphatic system, unlike the circulatory system, does not have a central pump like the heart to maintain its flow. Instead it relies on muscle contraction, stretching and skeletal motion to keep the lymph moving. You can help to stimulate the effective flow of lymph through exercise, stretching and massage. The neck, pelvis, arm pits and groin contain the greatest concentration of lymph nodes. These areas are the sites of the most bending, folding and stretching in the body, which facilitates the release of interstitial fluids and in turn drainage from the lymph nodes.

The circulatory and respiratory systems

When lymph enters the blood, substances that have to be excreted can be transported via the circulatory system. This is why strong and healthy circulation assists in the removal of waste. The blood carries toxins to the liver where further filtering takes place.

Our respiratory system releases excess carbon dioxide through the lungs. Fresh oxygen is also taken in by the lungs and put into circulation. The respiratory system can have an impact on body pH (acid/alkaline balance) and stimulate the relaxation response through shifts in blood chemistry in lung capillaries.

Physical exercise, which we will discuss later in this book, helps to support the lymphatic system as well as improving circulation and strengthening the heart. Maintaining good hydration also helps to support the body's ability to excrete toxins. Toxins are also released through the skin, as sweat.

The liver

Most toxins, both from our own cellular processes and from outside sources, are removed from the blood when it flows through the liver. The liver acts like a filter, removing toxins and packaging them for excretion. As well as filtering, the liver also transforms toxins into less toxic forms, which can be excreted through urine and faeces.

Filtering of blood is performed by kupffer cells, which are white blood cells found in the liver. These cells filter bacteria and antibodies as well as removing worn out red blood cells. In the process of removing old red blood cells, these white blood cells conserve the iron and discard the non-degradable portion in the form of bilirubin into the large intestine. From here it is excreted as a component of faeces. If the liver is overloaded with toxins, just as any filter can get clogged, the liver can become sluggish and its ability to perform its filtration role can become impaired. When this happens it potentially allows more antigens, bowel microorganisms and other toxins to remain in general circulation within the body.

Some toxins, including endocrine disruptors, are fat soluble and are transformed into a water soluble state through a series of complex chemical processes that take place in the liver. Once they become water soluble they can be excreted via the kidneys. This transformation process relies upon adequate resources coming from protein, vitamins and minerals. The optimal nutrition provided by the Fertility Code Nutrition Plan assists the liver in removing toxins from the body.

The kidneys

The main detoxification role of the kidneys is the production of urine. The average person has around 1.25 gallons of blood and the kidneys filter it continuously. The waste and water become urine, which is stored in the bladder prior to excretion. The kidneys also support the maintenance of the pH levels of our internal environment. Staying properly hydrated supports the healthy functioning of the kidneys.

The digestive system

Most digestion and nutrient absorption happens in the stomach and small intestine. After food has been ingested, the remains of indigestible food, mostly in the form of fibre, enter the colon, or large intestine. Digestion still occurs in the colon but not by the human body. Numerous colonies of bacteria live in the colon and break down and feed on these fibres. Many of these bacteria are beneficial, and by breaking down the fibres they provide nourishment for the colon and support immune function. However, the colon also plays host to harmful bacteria that secrete substances thought to interfere with the excretion of toxins and hence cause disease. These harmful bacteria tend to flourish when you provide them with some of the foods discouraged by the Fertility Code Nutrition Plan. Sticking to the plan helps to keep these harmful bacteria in check.

To enhance detoxification from the digestive system we want the journey of waste to the colon to happen fast but not too fast. When it is too slow constipation can occur and toxins end up being reabsorbed by the body. If the journey is too fast, diarrhoea may occur which can damage the beneficial intestinal flora, allowing harmful bacteria to thrive.

HOW DO YOU REDUCE TOXIC EXPOSURE?

Before you begin to remove toxins from your body you should first look at reducing your existing exposure to toxins. People respond to toxins in different ways and some of us can tolerate toxins for many years without experiencing any obvious repercussions. However, over time the toxic load increases and at some point you may find yourself suddenly affected, almost out of nowhere. How can this happen? Because our bodies are designed for survival, we develop a tolerance to these substances. However, even though we have developed initial tolerance, over time the toxins accumulate until their burden is too much for us to bear, and intolerance develops.

How toxic are you?

Ask yourself the following questions. The answers will give a clue as to what level of toxicity exists in your body.

- Do you experience fatigue and/or loss of energy and vitality?
- Do you experience swelling due to water retention?
- Do you have difficulty losing weight?
- Is there evidence of reduced immunity (e.g. frequent occurrence of colds and infections)?
- Do you frequently get headaches?
- Do you have allergies or sensitivities to foods or your environment?
- Do you suffer with sinus problems?
- Is your digestion sluggish or do you regularly experience heartburn, indigestion, stomach bloating or flatulence?
- Do you have constipation or diarrhoea?
- Do you smoke?
- Do you drink more than three units of alcohol a week?
- Do you notice a reduced ability to deal with stress or suffer with chronic anxiety?
- Do you suffer with chronic muscular or joint pain?
- Do you notice any impairment in your ability to think or concentrate?
- Do you suffer with premenstrual syndrome (PMS)?
- Do you use drugs – prescription or recreational – on a regular basis?

The chances are that most of us will answer yes to one or more of the above questions, which means that most of us should reduce our exposure to toxins. Of course the more yes answers you have the more likely it is that you are experiencing toxic overload.

In order to reduce toxic exposure you need to take things from the first step – awareness – to the next step, which is intervention. Some things you may not be able to change overnight. For example, it would be a mistake to stop taking prescription drugs without the approval and supervision of your doctor. However there are some toxic elements that you can safely eliminate.

Toxins you can proactively avoid

Artificial flavours, colours, preservatives and additives

Whilst these substances may be passed as safe for human consumption, the fact that they are artificial and not natural suggests that our bodies would be better off without them. I recommend eliminating these elements from your diet. The Fertility Code Nutrition Plan eliminates all these substances, as it avoids all processed foods. The rationale for avoiding consumption of artificial ingredients is quite straightforward: by avoiding artificial ingredients you are steering yourself towards nutrient rich, natural foods that are more likely to promote health and fertility.

Dairy

Cow's milk frequently contains added growth hormones and, in addition, the milk produced today contains the naturally present hormones of the female cow at a higher level than in years past. A recent study linked the consumption of cow's milk to higher incidence of hormone-related cancers. According to this review, milk from pregnant cows can contain up to 33 per cent more oestrogen than milk from a non-pregnant cow. (Ganmaa et al, 2005). Cows on dairy farms are kept pregnant so that they will provide a continual supply of milk.

Another study found that the level of oestrogen in processed milk, which contains the milk from both pregnant and non-pregnant cows, is generally on a par with raw milk from cows in the first and second trimester of pregnancy. The research concluded that a person's daily intake of oestrogen from milk is dramatically more than currently recognised (Malekinejad et al, 2006).

Genetically modified food

It is becoming increasingly more difficult to determine which foods have been genetically modified and which haven't. GM foods are a concern for overall health and fertility because commercially grown GM crops have been shown to contain pesticide residues of endocrine-disrupting chemicals at levels as high as 1,000 times the amount shown to exert biological effects. Until further long-term studies have been conducted on the safety of genetically modified food I recommend that you avoid them.

Alcohol

The relationship between alcohol and fertility was not clear until quite recently. Harvard researchers in 1994 found that women who were moderate drinkers – about one drink per day – experienced a slightly higher incidence of ovulatory infertility. However, when women drank more than one drink per day the risks were more dramatic. Endometriosis was found to be more common in women who drank, regardless of the amount. Both of these issues are linked to hormone function, which appears to be affected by alcohol intake.

In 1998 two further studies emphasised the negative effects of alcohol on fertility. A Danish study showed that women who drank moderately (fewer than five drinks a week) reduced their chances of conception, compared with women who didn't drink any alcohol. This study showed that the ability to become pregnant correlated directly with alcohol intake. Women who drank more than ten glasses of alcohol a week were found to be half as likely to become pregnant as those who drank fewer than five glasses a week.

Research at Johns Hopkins University in 1998 reinforced the Danish study and found that women who avoided both alcohol and caffeine were more than 250 per cent more likely to conceive than women who consumed alcohol and drank more than one cup of coffee a day. The highest conception rate was among women who didn't drink, didn't smoke, and didn't drink coffee.

Alcohol is clearly a factor when trying to conceive, but it is also a factor once you have conceived. According to some studies the risk of miscarriage increases even with moderate drinking during the early weeks of pregnancy, particularly in the first ten weeks. If a woman has just one glass of wine a day, her risk of miscarriage is twice that of a woman who doesn't drink at all. There have been other studies that have shown less conclusively that there is a link between alcohol and miscarriage, so further studies are necessary to establish the correct position on the issue. In the meantime, however, the best advice for women is to err on the side of caution and avoid all alcohol prior to conception and particularly in the first trimester of pregnancy.

As well as the possibility that moderate alcohol intake will increase ovulation problems and the risk of miscarriage, drinking two glasses of wine a day can have a detrimental effect on foetal development. An embryo can be affected by any toxin in the mother's system, especially during the first few weeks of its development, a time when you might not even realise that you are pregnant. Practically speaking, there is no safe level of alcohol intake during pregnancy.

Alcohol intake is not just damaging to female fertility; there is evidence that it can also have a significant impact on male fertility. Researchers have found that alcohol consumption produces changes in the shape of sperm and their ability to move. In men who drink heavily, the sperm production structure of the testicles can become damaged, so sperm count is affected.

The bottom line is that if you want to enhance your chances of conceiving, you should without question give up alcohol.

Caffeine in coffee and soft drinks

Many studies have established the negative impact coffee has on a woman's fertility. A 1997 report on more than 3,000 women in five European countries found that women who drink more than five cups of coffee (500 mg of caffeine) a day experienced delays in achieving conception. The Johns Hopkins research showed that drinking just one cup of coffee (100 mg) a day can have a negative impact on fertility. Most coffee today is sold in 250 ml cups which on average will contain 135 mg of caffeine.

But caffeine isn't just contained in coffee. You should take into consideration your total caffeine intake.

- A cup of take-out coffee – 135 mg of caffeine

- A cup of instant coffee – 65 mg of caffeine

- A cup of black tea – 30 mg of caffeine

- A cup of green tea – 30 mg of caffeine

- A cup of herbal tea – typically no caffeine

- A can of cola – 60 mg of caffeine

- A can of diet cola – 78 mg of caffeine

The Fertility Code Detox recommends that you limit your caffeine intake to 60 mg of caffeine or less a day.

Cigarettes

Quitting smoking has to be high on your priority list for detoxification, especially with regard to fertility. Smoking has strong associations with infertility. There are numerous reasons for this, including the increased levels of oxidative stress and the many toxic chemicals found in tobacco. A recent study found that women who smoke have higher levels of follicle stimulating hormone (FSH) during the first half of the menstrual cycle and higher levels of luteinising hormone (LH) during the second half of the menstrual cycle, which would indicate that the ovaries are not as responsive to reproductive hormones in smokers (Whitcomb et al, 2010).

A recent British study established a link between smoking and a higher rate of stillbirths, low birth weight babies, and sudden infant death syndrome (SIDS). A female smoker is less likely to achieve pregnancy through IVF when compared with a non-smoker. Smoking appears to accelerate the rate of egg loss, which might be what links smoking and reduced pregnancy rates following IVF. Women who smoke also have raised hormone levels, which indicates a depleted supply of eggs and prematurely aged follicles.

For men, smoking can lead to atherosclerosis, which can damage blood vessels and inhibit blood supply. This can ultimately cause impotence as a good supply and flow of blood is necessary to achieve an erection.

Drugs

Marijuana has been linked to loss of libido and impotence and to diminished fertility. It has also been associated with increased female hormones in men and the development of abnormally shaped sperm. This reduces the production of LH and therefore decreases the levels of testosterone in men. Male regular marijuana users experience ejaculation problems, poor sperm count and motility, together with loss of libido and impotence (Bari et al, 2011).

Cocaine is thought to have an impact on sperm development. Recent animal experiments have shown that it damages the cells that produce sperm.

Anabolic steroids, commonly used by men to build more muscular bodies, are also understood to have a negative impact on male fertility. These drugs can act as a male contraceptive by depressing normal hormone secretion and interfering with normal sperm production.

The good news is that in most cases when you stop using these substances, sperm production should eventually return to normal, although it may take a full seventy-four-day cycle of sperm production.

Solvents and pesticides

Numerous studies have shown a link between pesticides and chemical solvents in the environment with incidences of infertility in women and low sperm production and abnormal sperm in men. These substances are known as persistent organic pollutants (POPs) and they are compounds that do not degrade properly and have the potential to bio-accumulate in human tissue. POPs also include plastics and some pharmaceuticals. Frequent exposure to lawn and farm chemicals can be harmful, especially when they are sprayed where they can be inhaled or where they come into contact with the skin. When using any sort of weed killers or pesticides make sure to cover up as completely as possible, wearing a mask, trousers, long sleeves and vinyl gloves.

You should also wear similar protection when working with solvents such as paint thinners or turpentine and make sure that your working area has proper ventilation.

We can only do our best

Of course it is simply impossible to completely avoid exposure to all toxic chemicals; modern living puts us in direct contact with a number of harmful materials. When we eat foods that have been exposed to pesticides, additives and pollutants, we are ingesting toxic substances. Even when we eat organic food, there will still have been some pollution in the soil and air the food grew in. Our skin is also frequently exposed to chemicals in cosmetics, detergents and toiletries. The air we breathe is contaminated by car fumes, industrial waste and environmental pollutants.

So I am not suggesting that you must avoid all toxins as this is simply impractical. What I do suggest is that you are more aware of the toxins you encounter and that you take steps to sensibly minimise your exposure and hence the effects. It is difficult to say to what extent fertility problems are related to toxic exposure. We all have different genetic make-up and live in different environments, which makes it difficult for scientists to identify direct links between the many factors that relate to fertility and people's exposure to the very wide variety of toxic chemicals in existence. Nevertheless, the increased incidence of fertility related problems and the parallel increase in toxic chemicals suggest that limiting our toxic exposure and eliminating toxins as best we can, must become an important component of the Fertility Code.

DETOXING YOUR DIET

The dietary approach laid out in the Fertility Code Nutrition Plan is also the optimum approach to combating the toxins present in food and drink. By fully implementing the nutrition plan you are well on your way to achieving detoxification. Here, we will therefore focus on ways to approach implementing the nutrition plan.

Kitchen clear-out

Making dietary changes can be challenging and as a first step I highly recommend performing a kitchen clear-out. Out of sight means out of mind, and if you are hoping to avoid certain foods it makes no sense to have your fridge and cupboards full of these products. Give yourself plenty of time to perform the clear-out, and remember that clearing out does not mean consuming!

In order to do this correctly you may need to examine items one by one and look carefully at the ingredients list. So to begin your kitchen clear-out, remove the following foods from your kitchen:

The food detox list

- All canned food
- All processed food
- Anything containing MSG, artificial sweeteners, preservatives, flavourings and colourings
- Biscuits
- Breakfast cereals
- Butter
- Cakes
- Cheeses
- Chocolate
- Coffee
- Crisps
- Non free-range eggs
- Ice cream
- Jam and marmalade
- Margarine containing hydrogenated oil or trans fats
- Milk
- Popcorn
- Processed meats
- Red meat and pork
- Salt
- Salted nuts

↳ Sugar

↳ Sweets

↳ White bread

↳ White flour

Having removed the unhealthy foods from your kitchen cupboards and fridge, you can replace them with some of the healthy alternatives listed here.

FRIDGE-FREEZER	REPLACE WITH
Butter and margarine	Organic extra-virgin olive oil (store in cupboard)
Chicken nuggets	Organic free range chicken breasts
Chips	Organic sweet potato
Eggs	Organic free range eggs
Ice cream	Home-made ice-pops, made from 100 per cent fruit juice
Milk	Organic rice milk
Paté	Hummus
Processed meat and pork	Fish
Soft drinks	Fresh fruit juice
CUPBOARDS	**REPLACE WITH**
Biscuits	Fresh fruit
Cakes	Fresh fruit
Canned food	Fresh fruit and vegetables
Chocolate	Dried fruit (without additives)
Coffee	Green and herbal teas

Commercial breakfast cereal	Oatmeal and unsweetened, high fibre, low-salt cereal
Crisps	Unsalted nuts
Salt	Black pepper, garlic, dried herbs and spices
Salted nuts	Unsalted nuts
Stock cubes	Organic low-sodium stock cubes
Sugar	Organic honey
Sweets	Fruit and dried fruit (without additives)
Tea	Green and herbal teas
Tinned and instant soup	Home-made soup, made from organic vegetables
Tomato sauce	Freshly chopped tomatoes
White bread and rolls	Wholemeal bread
White flour	Wholegrain flour
White rice	Brown, basmati or wild rice

Detoxing your cooking utensils and storage jars

It is sensible to now continue your clear-out by removing utensils and other items that, when used in preparing or storing food, can lead to toxic contamination.

It is best to avoid all plastic-based packaging such as cling-film and plastic wrap. We now understand that the toxins found in plastic can also have hormone-mimicking properties and there is a suggestion that these could be linked to the rise of a number of reproductive disorders. Rather than wrapping fruit, vegetables and fish in plastic, use paper packaging instead.

The best materials for cooking with are glass, porcelain, earthenware, wood and stainless steel. Non-stick pans can emit toxins from their synthetic lining. Aluminium pots and pans can also release toxins.

Detoxing your cooking method

The best methods of cooking are stir-frying and steaming, as they ensure the retention of nutrients, vitamins and minerals.

Stir-frying – Mostly associated with Oriental cooking, stir-frying is one of the healthiest ways to cook and is an easy and quick method for cooking white meat, fish and vegetables. Stir-frying is done fast, over a high heat, with just the minimum amount of olive oil. The food is moved rapidly and continuously around the pan or wok to ensure equal distribution of heat. A sauce can be added at the end of the cooking process, and the ingredients can be allowed to briefly steam in the sauce.

Because of the speed of stir-frying there are few nutrients lost from the food. The vibrant colour of the food remains, which makes it more appealing to the eye. Typical stir-fry dishes contain just a small amount of meat or fish and relatively large quantities of vegetables, which is in line with the Fertility Code Nutrition Plan.

If you don't already have one, I would suggest that you purchase a stainless steel wok, which is a large, round-bottomed pan. Because of their shape, woks allow the ingredients to fall to the bottom of the pan, where the heat is the most intense. The classic round bottomed wok is designed for cooking over a flame, but you can also buy flat-bottomed woks for use on modern hobs.

Because you will be cooking very fast, it is important to prepare the ingredients before you start cooking. This includes having the correct amounts of sauces and seasonings to hand. You should cut vegetables into small pieces to allow for fast and even cooking. In Chinese medicine smaller pieces of food are understood to be easier to digest. Larger vegetables such as carrots are usually cut into strips or thinly sliced; round vegetables are cut into small pieces and broccoli and cauliflower are broken into florets. It is good to cut vegetables at an angle, as this exposes more of their surface area and they cook more quickly. Fish and poultry are usually diced or cut into thin strips or wafer-thin slices. Poultry, fish and tofu can be marinated for a few hours before cooking, as this helps to tenderise them as well as adding flavour.

When you have all your ingredients ready, you can begin cooking. Start by heating the wok and lightly drizzling olive oil around the edge. This oil will quickly heat up and coat the inside and bottom of the heated wok. When the wok is very hot you can start adding the ingredients. It is usual to add the flavouring ingredients, such as ginger or garlic, first, as these will flavour the oil, which will then transfer the flavours to the food. Then add the poultry, fish or thicker vegetables – whatever you are cooking that needs the longest time. Then add the remaining ingredients, obviously adding those that need the least cooking last. Toss and stir the ingredients with a wooden spatula throughout the cooking process, or gently shake the wok so the food keeps moving around. Adding sauce is usually the final step in the cooking process. Once the sauce has heated, the dish is ready to be served.

Steaming – This is another cooking method that has long been associated with Eastern cooking. It is one of the oldest cooking methods known, although it has had a surge in popularity in recent years. Steaming may even predate the discovery of fire, as it is believed that early man may have used stones from hot springs to cook food.

Steaming involves cooking food in the steam produced by boiling water. There are many steamers available – electrical steaming appliances, tiered pans with several steaming baskets, and petal steamers that open up to fit most saucepans and fold away for easy storage. In the East a bamboo steamer is often used. These are now available in the West, but the more usual method is to use a stainless steel, perforated basket placed on a saucepan.

Steaming is a light and very healthy cooking method, because mineral and vitamin loss is minimal, so valuable nutrients are preserved. As with stir-frying, the colours, flavours and textures of the food are retained, making the food pleasing to both the eye and the palate. Steaming also ensures that poultry and fish remain extremely tender.

To steam food:

✥ Position the steamer on a saucepan of boiling water

and fit the lid tightly so that the steam cannot escape. Once you have allowed steam to build up, add the ingredients to the basket.

↳ Make sure that the steamer basket isn't touching the water or else the food will be boiled rather than steamed.

↳ You can line the steamer with a muslin cloth to prevent delicate food from breaking up.

↳ Don't allow the pan to boil dry. You can keep a separate pot of boiling water close to hand should you need to replenish the water in the saucepan.

↳ Steaming doesn't add flavour, so if you wish you can marinade the food in advance, season it after cooking or serve it with a sauce.

↳ Serve the vegetables from the steamer as soon as the cooking time is up. If they are allowed to remain in the steamer they will continue to cook even after the heat is turned off, and they will go soggy, break apart and discolour.

♀♂

Of course there are other cooking methods, but they are less healthy than stir-frying and steaming; I would suggest that these methods should dominate your cooking. In particular you should avoid any method that requires you to use large amounts of oil or fat. Try to avoid overcooking as this has the potential to rob your food of vital minerals and vitamins. There are two cooking methods that I particularly discourage because I think that they present health risks.

Microwaves

Microwave cooking robs your food and hence your body of vital nutrients and as such it must be avoided. Microwaving is a relatively new form of cooking that can hardly be described as natural. Microwaves can be found in most homes, unfortunately. I say unfortunately because not only does food cooked in a microwave taste – in my opinion – not quite right, but it is proven to deplete the nutritional value of the food. More importantly, microwaves also pose a risk to long-term health.

When food is cooked by other methods, heat moves from outside to inside the food. With microwave cooking the reverse happens; food is cooked from within and a process takes place that can alter its chemical structure. The microwaves that bombard the food cause molecules to rotate millions of times a second. The structure of these molecules is literally deformed by this process and new, unnatural compounds are created. These compounds can be difficult for your body to deal with. In addition, vitamins, minerals and proteins are damaged and food can lose its bio-availability, which means that you will be less likely to absorb nutrients from it.

There is also the danger of exposure to harmful electromagnetic radiation from the microwave itself. If you have a microwave, my advice is to stop using it, or better still, throw it out as part of the kitchen clear-out.

Barbecues

There are numerous health issues surrounding barbecuing food. First of all, there is the potentially carcinogenic smoke, containing benzopyrene, that is produced when you grill meat over charcoal. Then there are heterocyclic amines (HCAs), which are formed when meats are cooked at very high temperatures until they char. There is evidence indicating that HCAs are carcinogenic. Researchers from the National Cancer Institute in the US have identified a link between stomach cancer and meats cooked until charred. There is also evidence that the high smoke intake of barbecued meat is associated with an increased risk of developing colorectal, pancreatic and breast cancer; a German study revealed that women who frequently ate barbecued food had double the risk of developing breast cancer compared with women who never ate barbecued food.

Putting it simply, you should avoid eating barbecued food.

♀♂

IMPLEMENTING THE FERTILITY CODE DETOX

It is a powerful asset that our body is designed to both deal with toxins and to repair itself once toxins have been removed. We have already looked at the various toxins that can have an impact on your health and fertility. Now we will address how to change behaviours and lifestyle choices to help boost your fertility.

The Fertility Code Detox works on the following principles:

1. A primary cause of illness is the accumulation of unnecessary waste, resulting in poison retention, ill health and fertility problems.

2. Your body is designed to support optimal function and gives signals when these toxins are introduced to your body.

3. Given the proper environment, your body has the power to heal itself and return to its normal healthy state.

Conquering food cravings: the Revulsion Technique

Changing your diet is challenging. Foods that have been a central part of your diet for many years can often feel like part of who you are. When I changed my own diet back in 1998, following my diagnosis with multiple sclerosis, I changed it completely, literally overnight. There are foods that were a regular part of my diet that I have never eaten since. I did experience food cravings; I felt pangs and yearnings for sugar in the form of sweet food. For as long as I could remember I had eaten enormous amounts of cheese, and it was the first food I would turn to for a savoury snack. However, I used a number of methods to ensure a relatively easy and rapid transition to a clean diet. Shortly after overcoming the initial cravings, I felt such a huge benefit to my health that remaining on course became easy.

I used very effective mental techniques to manage my cravings. Whenever I felt I needed to eat sweet food or sugar I imagined the harmful bacteria and cells – the kind of things that had lived off this sugar – creating discomfort for me in an effort to encourage me to feed them this sugar again and keep them alive. They were beginning to starve and the harsher my cravings were, the closer I felt I was to gaining victory over the harmful bacteria. This mental technique worked a treat. Making such a radical change may seem difficult, but I am convinced that doing it this way is more effective than making partial or gradual changes. When your goals are vague or blurred your mind becomes less clear about what you are attempting to achieve; as a result you are more likely to fail. There are numerous methods you can use to support rapid changes in your eating habits and make an effective transition to your new healthy eating regime. Perhaps the most powerful of these methods involves the use of mental revulsion.

You might forget this, but many foods that become addictive are often unpleasant to taste when you initially encounter them. Just as the first time someone smokes they usually feel nauseous, the first time we encounter harmful foods, our body frequently rejects the taste. However, because of our own persistence and the mental conditioning of advertisements promoting the products, we manage to train our bodies to accept these foods.

The revulsion technique is based on relearning what our bodies already knew in the first place – that these foods are not good for us. We simply train ourselves to remember what it feels like to be disgusted when we consume these foods.

So, imagine a dead rat lying at the side of the road, with its belly split open and its guts spilled out. Hundreds of maggots are feeding on the juicy entrails. Now imagine someone picks the rat up, slices off a cross section and uses it to make a hamburger. The more clearly you create this image in your mind, the less inclined you will be to want to eat a hamburger.

Obviously the burger is not made from rat meat and you might think it is unfair to impose revulsion of something that is completely unrelated to the product. However, this is simply the reverse of the same technique used by advertisers every single day. Eating greasy, salty, sugary food does not make life extraordinarily exciting or glamorous, nor does it make you more attractive to the opposite sex. Advertisers frequently use completely unrelated images and ideas to create feelings about the products they are selling. Have you noticed how many advertisers use comedians for their voiceovers? We are used to experiencing laughter and enjoyment when we hear a famous comedian's voice. When that comedian provides a voiceover, at a subconscious level we transfer this sense of joy and happiness to the product. Despite the fact that we are consciously aware that these foods will harm our health and make us fat, we are fooled into feeling that the products will make us happy, surround us with friends and even make us more attractive.

Our thinking becomes distorted and we become obsessed with the search for comfort and pleasure and forget the many harmful effects. Before long it is the junk-food manufacturers who are in control of our minds and our lives. As we dance to their tune like puppets on a string, we develop a host of warning signs that we overlook – gas, obesity, bloating, indigestion, skin problems and illness – but we continue to fool ourselves that we have exercised choice.

The closer we are to experiencing pleasure, the more we become obsessed with it. We focus exclusively on the pleasure and decide that we need it. Just as a drug addict focuses on the pleasure of feeding his craving, whilst ignoring the detrimental effects on his health, the waste of money, the pain of withdrawal and the harmful effects on friends and family. If he could look at the complete picture, he would not contemplate using drugs. Similarly with junk foods, if we forced ourselves to look at the entire picture, we would never eat them at all.

We usually try to combat compulsive or comfort eating in the moments just before eating. This is the least effective time to fight the compulsion. Just as you should never go shopping for food when you are hungry, you should also carefully choose the time when you are going to conquer food compulsions, and it should be a time when you are relaxed and feel good.

The Revulsion Effect

The Revulsion Effect is a powerful tool to help you to stop eating harmful foods. It shuts off the pleasure tape and creates the opportunity for you to refocus on what you really want. It will allow you to jump out of the obsession cycle and give you the opportunity to look at the importance of your overall health and fertility goal.

The Revulsion Effect begins by creating a feeling of nausea. You can try this now. The first time you may have to focus intently on an imagined dead rat or a greasy hair in your soup, but with just a little practice you can create this revulsion effect easily and at will. Use it frequently in the beginning. At home or in the supermarket, pick up a product, create revulsion, put the product back and move on. Use this method several times a day for a week, and it soon becomes a powerful tool.

Then, when you are tempted by bad foods, simply call upon the feeling of revulsion by focusing on something that makes you feel nauseous and say to yourself, 'I don't feel like having any of this food.' Leave the shop or kitchen and get moving. There is no battle of will, no fighting any obsession, just one moment of feeling nausea and off you go. Each time you conquer a food craving, you will become stronger and defeating that craving will be even easier the next time.

When to use the Revulsion Effect

- When you are not hungry but are thinking about food
- When you are shopping and want to avoid purchasing junk food
- When you overeat
- Whilst visualising the foods you are trying to quit eating

Revulsion exercise

- **Step one** – Consider a food or drink unhelpful to fertility that you have experienced cravings for. Let's use coffee as an example. Now close your eyes and see a mug of coffee in front of you. Allow the feelings to come to you as if you were just about to taste the coffee.

- **Step two** – Now imagine a drink or liquid that you find disgusting, something that makes you feel nauseous, perhaps a glass of rotten raw eggs. With your eyes still closed, imagine mixing this drink with the coffee you are craving. Visualise the rotten egg yolks sluggishly plopping into the coffee.

- **Step three –** Now see yourself drinking the mixture and feel the gut-wrenching sensation of the rotten egg yolk sliding down your throat.

- Do you feel like drinking coffee now? Practise this again and again and with other foods that are unhelpful to your fertility. Your feelings towards these foods will quickly begin to change.

Sample revulsion thoughts

- Crisps – Visualise old, parasite-ridden mouldy potatoes being sliced and dipped in two-week-old, already-used fat.

- Margarine – Imagine a factory worker filling the plastic tub while snot drips from his nose into the container, mixing with the margarine.

- Red meat – Visualise a terrified animal screaming as it is being slaughtered and see yourself gorging on the animal flesh, still warm from the slaughter.

- Milk – Visualise suckling on a cow's udder

The Fertility Code Environmental Detox

When you think of pollution, you typically think of industrial chimney smoke or a polluted urban area. However it is likely that some of the most harmful and toxic pollutants are found in your home. Because of our regular proximity to these pollutants we tend not to notice them even though they potentially do more harm than any smoke-belching factory.

Whilst it is impossible to avoid all toxic chemicals, you can dramatically decrease your exposure by simply paying close attention to the products you use in your household, garden and on your body. It may again involve a clear-out and making certain changes, but you will soon see and feel the benefits. The following are key steps for detoxing your environment:

✤ Remove all tobacco and tobacco products from your home. If any of your friends or family smoke, encourage them to do so outside, or better still encourage them to quit. As second-hand tobacco smoke contains over four thousand chemicals, many of which are undoubtedly unhelpful to your fertility and some of which are carcinogenic, there is no place for smoking in your home. If you are the one producing these chemicals by smoking, then follow the Fertility Code Nicotine Detox.

✤ Clear out your domestic cleaning products that contain toxic chemicals. Consider healthier alternatives such as vinegar and water for cleaning windows, lemon juice for cleaning dishes and bathroom areas, and baking soda and water for cleaning ovens. Undiluted white vinegar can be used as a household disinfectant. A number of environmentally safe cleaning products are now on the market. The Ecover brand produces cleaning products that can be safely used in your home.

✤ Throw out all artificial air fresheners. Although they may smell pleasant, they frequently emit substances such as ethanol, formaldehyde, phenol and xylene. Many of these are reproductive toxins and can cause both male and female infertility. As an alternative, use proper ventilation together with natural essential oils and flowers.

✤ When using scented candles, make sure that they are made from plant wax and beeswax and that they contain only pure essential oils and not synthetic fragrances.

✤ Remember to use your kitchen extractor fan and make sure that it is vented outside.

↻ Avoid exposure to all products that contain methylene chloride and benzene. Methylene chloride is found in paint strippers and aerosol spray paint and reports suggest it may inhibit sperm production. A study of women working in a pharmaceutical factory found an increased risk of spontaneous abortions associated with exposure to several chemicals, including methylene chloride. Women working with glue were found to have methylene chloride in the foetal tissues. This indicates methylene chloride crosses the placental barrier. Men exposed to benzene at levels close to the permissible limit are more likely to have an abnormal number of chromosomes in their sperm, researchers reported in the journal *Environmental Health Perspectives*. Some sperm can develop with either too many or too few chromosomes. Known as aneuploidy, this can have an adverse impact on fertility and foetal development. Aneuploidy (in either the sperm or the egg) is the largest known cause of miscarriage.

↻ Bring plants into your home as they combat air pollution, but remember to remove them from your bedroom at nighttime, when plants generally absorb oxygen and release carbon dioxide.

The Fertility Code Skincare Detox

We all want to look our best, but most of us don't realise that many of the skincare products we use are loaded with chemicals that are potentially harmful to fertility. Perfumes, make-up, deodorants and shampoos often contain toxins that are harmful to our bodies. A notable benefit of The Fertility Code Detox is that you are far less likely to need many of these products to enhance your appearance. Detoxification will improve your skin naturally.

↻ Choose only cosmetics and skincare products that are chemical-free and safe.

↻ Avoid the overuse of perfumes and colognes. These

are frequently made from petrochemicals and other synthetic toxic materials. Choose organic perfumes where possible.

 ֍ There are now a variety of non-toxic, plant-based and biodegradable hair colourants available. If you do colour your hair, use these natural products.

 ֍ Avoid using commercial deodorants and antiperspirants. These products frequently contain harmful ingredients such as aluminium and triclosan. Aluminium is believed to be detrimental to fertility and recent findings raise strong concerns about triclosan's possible effects on foetal growth and development (Giudice et al, 2006). There is an emerging body of research that suggests triclosan is an endocrine disruptor and should be eliminated from consumer products.

The Fertility Code Nicotine Detox

If you smoke, quitting is one of the most important things you can do to enhance fertility and improve the outcomes of pregnancy. Women who smoke have significantly lower levels of oestrogen, which could lead to problems in conceiving. It can also cause an early menopause. In men, smoking decreases sperm count and motility, increases the number of abnormal sperm, and reduces testosterone levels. Smoking causes so much direct damage to your body that kicking this habit must be given priority. Why would you start eating pure and healthy food and continue to inhale literally thousands of toxic chemicals into your lungs?

How to quit smoking

The Fertility Code offers some powerful techniques that you can utilise to remove nicotine from your life for good. If you are hoping to achieve pregnancy that should easily provide the initial motivation you need to conquer smoking. Use all of these techniques regularly and you will soon see the health and fertility benefits of being a non-smoker.

The benefits of quitting cigarettes

Within twenty minutes of smoking that last cigarette, your body begins a series of changes that continue for years.

Twenty minutes after quitting – Your heart rate and blood pressure drop to a level close to that before your last cigarette. The temperature of your hands and feet increases, returning to normal.

Twelve hours after quitting – The carbon monoxide level in your blood drops to normal. The oxygen level in your blood increases to normal.

Twenty-four hours after quitting – Your heart attack risk begins to drop.

Forty-eight hours after quitting – Your nerve endings start re-growing and your ability to smell and taste is enhanced.

Two weeks to three months after quitting – Your lung function improves by up to 30 per cent and your circulation improves.

One to nine months after quitting – Cilia regrow in the lungs, increasing your ability to handle mucus, cleaning your lungs and lowering your risk of lung infections. Your lungs begin functioning better and overall energy increases.

One year after quitting – Your added risk of coronary heart disease is half that of a smoker.

Five years after quitting – Your stroke risk is reduced to that of someone who has never smoked.

In preparation for quitting, do the following:

1. Tell friends and family members that you are quitting and ask for their support and encouragement. Once you ask for support you'll be surprised how much it can help and how much motivation it provides for you to succeed.

2. Ask friends and family members not to smoke in your presence. Don't be afraid to ask. This is more important than you may realise.

3. On your quit day, hide all ashtrays and destroy all cigarettes.

4. For the first few days, drink lots of water and fluids to help flush out the nicotine and other poisons from your body.

5. If there are any places in particular where you used to smoke, change the layout of these places. Move the seats, or change the location of the phone. Our brains create a lot of associations around smoking and these should be destroyed as much as possible by making these changes.

Technique one

Deep breathing is perhaps the most powerful technique for anyone who is stopping smoking. People often mistakenly believe that they relax when smoking because of nicotine. People do relax when they smoke, not because of nicotine but rather because of taking time out and breathing deeply. If you feel cravings for a cigarette, do the following exercise three times.

1. Inhale your deepest breath and fill your lungs. Then, very gently, exhale. Purse your lips so that the air comes out very slowly.

2. As you exhale, close your eyes and let your chin gradually sink onto your chest. Visualise all the tension leaving your body, slowly draining out of your fingers and toes, just flowing out.

You can use this technique when you find yourself craving a cigarette in stressful situations. The best thing is that every time you succeed with the technique its power increases.

Technique two

Get a sheet of paper and write down the six main reasons from the following list why you don't like smoking, why it is bad and why you have stopped.

1. Women smokers take longer to conceive when compared with non-smokers. This is also true if you are a passive smoker.

2. Smoking makes your breath, hair and clothes stink.

3. Miscarriage rates are higher in women who smoke compared with non-smokers.

4. One in five die from illnesses directly linked to smoking.

5. Menopause occurs earlier in female smokers.

6. If you smoke regularly for a long time, you may get a disease called peripheral vascular disease. This disease causes narrowing of the blood vessels, which restricts blood flow to the hands, feet and of course the reproductive organs. This can lead to gangrene and amputation of limbs.

7. There is an increased risk of an ectopic pregnancy (pregnancy in the fallopian tube) in smokers.

8. Smoking messes with your body chemistry. It decreases the levels of vitamin C in the blood, for example. Vitamin C, among other things, protects you against carcinogens, boosts immunity and helps prevent heart disease. Smoking increases cholesterol. It's estimated that every cigarette you smoke raises your total cholesterol by about half a point.

9. Male smokers have a 17 per cent reduction in their number of sperm compared with male non-smokers.

10. Smokers have a higher frequency of severe depression, anxiety disorders and other psychological problems.

11. Smoking depletes male hormones, and the risk of

impotence is about 50 per cent for male smokers in their thirties or forties.

12. Smoking causes cancer. The links between cigarettes and cancer of the oral cavity, oesophagus, lungs, kidneys, pancreas, stomach, cervix and bladder are indisputable.

13. Male smokers have decreased sperm quality and increased presence of fragmented DNA.

14. If you smoke, you have an increased risk of gum disease, muscle injury, angina, neck pain, back pain, abnormal eye movements, circulatory disease, fungal eye infection, ulcers, osteoporosis, cataracts, Crohn's disease, pneumonia, depression, psoriasis, type-two diabetes, skin wrinkling, hearing loss, flu, rheumatoid arthritis, and many other conditions.

Technique three

Next, we are going to use a revulsion technique to reprogramme your mind to feel disgusted by cigarettes. Recall four times when you thought to yourself, *I've got to quit smoking*, or when you felt disgusted by smoking. Maybe somebody you know was badly affected by smoking. Take a moment now to remember four separate occasions when you felt that you had to quit or were disgusted by smoking.

Close your eyes and remember each one of these four times as if they are happening right now. Jump from one memory to another and keep going through each until you can make them as vivid as possible. See what you saw, hear what you heard and feel what you felt. Try to associate a separate single word with each memory. Now scroll through each word, quickly recalling each of those memories over and over, again and again. Rapidly overlap each memory with the next until you feel totally and utterly disgusted by cigarettes and smoking.

Technique four

Have you ever heard of an adult who continues to carry a security blanket that they had as a baby? The human mind is very sensitive to associations, and in this case the person as an infant associated comfort and safety with the blanket. Subconsciously they have tricked themselves into believing that this sense of comfort has emanated from the blanket itself.

In a similar way, people become accustomed to cigarettes in certain situations. If you smoked when with friends or taking time out you fooled yourself into thinking that the enjoyment of being with friends or taking a break is due to the cigarette. This is of course as delusional as the blanket being a source of safety. So, now that you have quit smoking, continue to give yourself relaxation times but do something different. Go for a walk or chat with a friend.

IN SUMMARY

- ✤ Clear out your kitchen and use the Revulsion Technique to help implement your nutrition plan.

- ✤ Use healthier cooking methods as well as cooking materials that do not expose you unnecessarily to toxic residues.

- ✤ Cigarette smoke is one of the most significant causes of fertility problems, so avoid exposure to second hand smoke.

- ✤ If you are the one who is smoking, now is the time to free yourself of this harmful habit. Use the techniques in this chapter to give up nicotine for good.

- ✤ Avoid exposure to harmful chemical toxins by avoiding products that contain them.

- ✤ Having addressed your exposure to harmful toxins, your body is turbo charged to become more fertile. Continuing to fuel your body with foods of the Fertility Code Nutrition Plan will support your recovery. But just as stagnant waters become unhealthy, our bodies – which are mostly water – also need to keep moving. This leads us to the final element of the Fertility Code - the optimum exercise to enhance your fertility.

Optimal EXERCISE
for Fertility

"If we could give every person the right amount of nourishment and exercise, not too little and not too much, we would have found the surest way to health"

Hippocrates

INTRODUCTION

We all know that exercise plays an important role in maintaining health and well-being, but it also plays a significant role in improving fertility. Exercise can help you to reach and maintain your ideal weight, reduce stress and improve blood flow to your reproductive system. All of these things can improve your fertility, both directly and indirectly. This will come as no surprise to most people, as we generally associate exercise with good health. However, it might surprise you to know that too much exercise can also stress your body, impede ovulation and drastically reduce fertility. To increase your chances of having a baby you should certainly exercise, but only the appropriate exercise and the right amount.

BENEFITS OF EXERCISE

Exercise improves your blood circulation and endocrine function and therefore helps to regulate hormone levels. One key hormone on which exercise has an effect is cortisol – the stress hormone. Exercise reduces the body's production of cortisol and so reduces stress, one of the main stumbling blocks to fertility.

Regular exercise also helps to keep your metabolic system healthy. Being inactive can cause your cells to become insensitive to insulin, which can lead to raised blood-sugar levels. Chronic high blood-sugar levels can contribute to ovulation problems and therefore impede conception. It is also important to maintain control over blood-sugar levels during pregnancy.

A study published in 2007 in *Obstetrics and Gynecology* followed

17,544 women who were trying to get pregnant over a period of eight years. The study revealed that regular physical exercise combined with a healthy diet and weight control reduced the risk of infertility by 69 per cent. This suggests that exercise is beneficial, although it is difficult to distinguish from this study which benefits accrue because of exercise and which are due to healthy eating.

Benefits of exercise before and during pregnancy

- Better sense of emotional well-being
- Reduced stress levels
- Improved circulation
- Enhanced sleep
- Improved tolerance to pregnancy discomfort
- Better recovery rate after the baby is born
- Better weight management

WEIGHT MANAGEMENT

One of the main reasons why you would wish to exercise is to achieve better weight management. About 12 per cent of fertility issues are associated with weight problems. Studies have shown that having a body fat level of just 10 per cent above or below normal can have a significant impact on fertility. Around 30 per cent of the oestrogen in a woman's body is produced by fat cells. Having too many or too few of these fat cells can cause hormonal imbalances. Being overweight can elevate oestrogen levels, which can in turn impair ovulation. Being overweight can also increase the amount of insulin you produce. For women this can cause the ovaries to produce more male hormones and prevent ovulation. The goal of the Fertility Code is to make sure that you achieve pregnancy at the lowest-risk weight range. Achieving optimum weight will reduce your chances of encountering weight-related pregnancy complications. As a first step you need to determine where you are in relation to your ideal body weight. To do this we use a measure called the Body Mass Index (BMI). Your BMI is a relationship between your height and your weight and provides a simple measure of a person's 'thickness'. A frequent use of BMI is to assess how much an individual's body weight departs from what is normal for a person of his or her height. The weight excess or deficiency is usually accounted for by body fat or lack of it, although other factors, such as muscularity, also affect BMI.

BMI levels for overweight and obesity are set by the World Health Organization (WHO), which defines overweight as a BMI equal to or more than 25, and obesity as a BMI equal to or more than 30. The chart at the end of this chapter will help you determine what your BMI is.

BMI is calculated by multiplying your weight in pounds by 703 and then dividing that number by your height in inches squared. For example, if you are 5 ft 8", this is a total of 68". The square of 68 is 68 x 68, or 4,624. If your weight is 150 lbs, you multiply that by 703 and you get 105,450. Dividing 4,624 into 105,450 generates a BMI 22.8. This is within the normal adult range.

BMI

Underweight	Below 18.5
Normal	18.5 – 24.9
Overweight	25.0 – 29.9
Obese	30.0 – 39.9
Morbidly obese	40.0 and above

If your BMI falls within the normal range you will be at the lowest risk for encountering many health- and pregnancy-related problems. If you are in this range you also have significantly more favourable odds of both conceiving and delivering a healthy baby. A study carried out by researchers at the Academic Medical Center in the Netherlands showed that overweight and obese women experience sub-fertility even when they ovulate. Sub-fertility means that there is less chance of becoming pregnant, even though you may not be suffering from infertility. In other words a woman with a regular cycle and no obvious fertility problems may still encounter difficulty getting pregnant if she is overweight. The study also showed that the more overweight the woman is, the lower her chances are of pregnancy. For every BMI unit over 29, chance of pregnancy fell by 4 per cent. Severely obese women, with BMI's of 35 to 40, had up to a 43-per-cent lower chance of achieving pregnancy compared with women with a BMI below 29. Also women who become pregnant at a normal weight reduce their risk of pregnancy complications such as gestational diabetes. If you have a BMI of between 25 and 29.9 before pregnancy, you have double the chance of developing this condition, whilst a BMI over 30 triples your risk.

What about men?

A Danish study found that overweight or obese men have significantly lower sperm counts than men of normal weight. The study revealed that sperm concentration was nearly 22 per cent lower in overweight men and that sperm count was 24 per cent lower, compared with healthy-weight men.

RECOMMENDED APPROACH TO WEIGHT REDUCTION BEFORE PREGNANCY

So we know that being overweight makes it harder to conceive. If you do conceive complications are more likely to happen if you are overweight. Therefore it makes sense for a woman to set a target-weight goal and try to achieve this gradually even before you try to get pregnant. The following are the key approaches to healthy weight reduction:

- Try to lose between 1 and 2 lbs per week and not any more than this. This gradual weight loss will mean that you are more likely to lose mostly fat, rather than muscle. When you lose weight faster than this, you are likely to be losing muscle mass and water. This can be unhelpful and can interfere with hormonal balance, making it harder to conceive.

- Follow the Fertility Code Nutrition Plan. You should avoid fad diets and weight-loss products which can often interfere with your chances of conceiving.

- Don't skip meals. Make sure to have a healthy and

hearty breakfast every morning. This will make you less likely to be tempted by cravings in mid morning.

℘ Exercise plays an important role in losing weight and you should build regular physical activity into your daily routine by following the exercise recommendations in this chapter. If you have not been exercising before now, be patient with your body and work towards your target weight at a slow steady pace. Moderate exercise performed on a daily basis supported by a healthy eating plan is the key to achieving your target weight.

℘ Weigh yourself no more than once or twice a week and pay more attention to how your clothes fit.

℘ Drink water regularly throughout the day.

℘ Recognise that sometimes your weight will plateau. This is a normal part of steady weight loss. If this continues for more than a few weeks look again at your food and drink intake. Even occasional slips from your nutrition plan can be enough to hinder progress with weight reduction.

♀♂

DRAWBACKS OF TOO MUCH EXERCISE

So if you're looking to improve your health and fertility, you might assume exercising is one of the best actions to take. Whilst this is true, it is not the full story. With exercise, too much of a good thing can be bad.

It might seem illogical, but women who regularly exercise for four or more hours per week reduce their fertility. This is evidenced by a study that showed that women who take this much exercise are 40 per cent less likely to have success with IVF than those who do not exercise at all. How can this be? Well if we look to the East we might have the answer. Whilst the Western mindset equates fitness with health, as if they are synonymous, Eastern medicine recognises that too much strenuous exercise can be bad for you. Strenuous exercise actually strains the body, and although it can make you very fit in terms of sporting performance, when carried out over a sustained period it can be detrimental to health and fertility. Research suggests that excessive exercise can put stress on a woman's reproductive system, which makes her body 'protect' itself from pregnancy. Mark Hornstein, the lead researcher at Brigham and Women's Hospital in Boston, where these studies took place, said that this might be explained by the subtle hormonal changes caused by exercise.

In a Harvard Medical School study, the health of over 5,300 athletic women was evaluated and they found that the strenuous exercise associated with competitive sports seemed to impair fertility. These athletes frequently presented with an absence of menstruation and ovulation. So, women dedicated to elite sporting performance who want to have a baby should consider cutting back on the amount of exercise they do, or discontinue their workout programmes altogether.

Women who exercise excessively can become underweight or have too little body fat. This can result in an oestrogen deficiency and can hamper menstruation and inhibit ovulation. Although the woman may have plenty of healthy eggs in her ovaries, they may not be released due to this hormonal deficiency. Women who exercise too much have also been shown to have raised levels of the stress hormone, cortisol, in their bodies. We know that this can also impair ovulation as well as interfere with the implantation of a fertilised egg.

What should be noted from the Harvard study, however, is that the women evaluated were highly athletic and almost all would have been classified as having average or below average body fat. Many women encountering fertility issues are not so athletic and therefore it doesn't necessarily follow that everyone should cut down on or eliminate exercise. It's about achieving a balance.

Case study – Andrea and David

Andrea and David had been trying to conceive for almost a year without success when they came to the clinic. They both had busy office jobs, which meant that they had little time for exercise and their food choices were rarely good. They were now at the stage where they were considering medical treatment, but they already realised that they needed to address their lifestyle. Both Andrea and David were overweight and they agreed to implement the Fertility Code Nutrition Plan supported by regular exercise. The aim was that they would lose between 1 and 2 lbs a week until they reached their optimal BMI's. At the recommended pace this took them just over three months to achieve. After four months they reported improved sense of well-being, better sleep and more energy. But more importantly they were also able to report that Andrea had become pregnant during their third month of following the plan. Later that year they became proud parents of a baby boy, Jack.

Men and over-exercise

It seems that men can work out more than women without adversely affecting their fertility. However, men also need to be careful. Men who over-exercise may also become underweight, which can have an impact on sperm motility and can also cause abnormal sperm morphology. Exercising too much can cause the internal temperature of a man's testicles to become too high, which can lead to sperm death and low sperm count.

Long-distance runners, who are frequently very lean, may

experience fertility problems due to a combination of high-level exercise and little body fat. Studies have also shown that cycling for long periods on a bicycle can flatten the artery that controls blood flow to the penis. This can cause nerve damage and it is recommended that cyclists switch from a solid bicycle seat to one that has an oval opening in the saddle.

♀♂

RECOMMENDED APPROACH TO WEIGHT GAIN BEFORE PREGNANCY

If your body weight is too low, now is the right time to get to the optimum weight to achieve and support a healthy pregnancy. For many people it is hard to imagine putting on weight as being a challenge. But the key point here is that we want you to achieve this in a healthy way that will enhance your fertility. This would not be achieved by eating junk food and taking no exercise.

Try to gain between 1 and 2 lbs per week and not any more than this. Eating about 500 extra calories per day should add an additional pound to your weight each week. Aim to get these additional calories by eating more food recommended by the Fertility Code Nutrition Plan.

Make sure that you are not skipping meals. Continue to follow the Fertility Code Nutrition Plan but don't wait until you are hungry before eating. As well as eating three balanced meals a day make a conscious effort to snack between meals. These snacks should be healthy options such as nuts, dried fruit, fresh fruit, fruit juices etc.

Include high fibre food as part of your diet. Make sure to also drink plenty of water and fruit juice so that you don't feel too full or even constipated.

Whilst physical activity is helpful for improving emotional well-being, it is not helpful for weight gain. Limit your exercise to very moderate activity that does not burn too many calories.

After you have achieved your weight gain target keep track by weighing yourself once a week. If you begin to lose weight again make sure to follow the guidelines as described above to regain weight.

GETTING THE BALANCE RIGHT

> ### Case study – Barry
>
> Barry and his wife had been trying to conceive for six months when they visited the clinic. A semen analysis had revealed that Barry's sperm count was low and they hoped that acupuncture might be able to help. During the initial consultation Barry spoke of his fanaticism for triathlons and fitness in general. He had always been very healthy and it had come as a shock to him that his fertility was anything less than perfect. However, it was clear that the intensity of Barry's training was putting huge pressure on his body. It took time for him to get his head around this. For him fitness equalled health, but I explained how extreme fitness could also mean extreme physical strain. As difficult as it was for him, he agreed to reduce the intensity of his training. The semen analysis was repeated four months later and this time the count was within normal range. Shortly after this Barry and his wife told me they were expecting their first baby. Barry was back competing in triathlons soon after that.

So should you exercise or not? How do you get it right? Like many things regarding health and fertility, the secret is down to that key word – balance. We must look at exercise within an overall context of creating a healthy lifestyle. Moderation is the key to exercise if you are trying to conceive. If you are overweight and just beginning an exercise programme, start slowly and think of it as a long-term plan that you will stick to.

Planning your exercise

Exercising gently but regularly will give you the most benefit. Make sure to drink plenty of water before, during and after exercise. If you have not exercised before, make sure that you consult your doctor prior to starting. It is important to dress appropriately and to wear loose-fitting, comfortable clothing.

The recommended amount of exercise you should take depends to a large degree on your body weight. If your BMI is below average you should restrict your exercise to the very minimum. In this context your goal should be to gain weight. Exercise is not conducive to weight gain and consequently it must be curtailed. If you are underweight, limit yourself to a maximum of just fifteen minutes of gentle exercise per day. Go for a gentle stroll or perform some gentle chi gong.

You should also consider keeping exercise to a minimum if any of the following apply to you:

- Cardiac problems
- Asthma or chronic respiratory problems
- High blood pressure
- Muscle or joint problems
- History of premature labour
- History of repeated miscarriages
- Expecting twins or multiples
- Persistent bleeding

If your BMI is within the normal range, you can increase the time you spend exercising to approximately thirty minutes per day. You should always aim to avoid overheating and only perform low-impact exercise such as gentle walking, yoga, chi gong and swimming. If you are overweight, you should exercise for between forty-five and sixty minutes per day and you can add some higher-intensity exercise such as cycling. The exercise should remain low impact, however, and you should feel good afterwards. If you feel exhausted after exercise, you either did too much or the intensity was too high.

Listen to your body when you are exercising. If something hurts or does not feel right, you should stop. Other stop signs include:

- Dizziness
- Headaches
- Shortness of breath

♮ Heart palpitations

♮ Heavy sweating

Safety guidelines for exercise

Whether you are very fit or just starting to exercise, it is a good idea to understand the manner in which you should progress to fitness. It takes about three or four months for an unfit person to achieve a healthy level of fertility fitness when starting from scratch. Exercise must be gentle and you should avoid muscle strains. Your heart and lungs will adapt to exercise within a month. To prevent injuries follow these recommendations:

1. Include a five-minute gentle warm-up as part of your exercise routine. Walking at a slow and comfortable pace is an ideal way to do this. At the end of your workout perform a similar five-minute gentle cool-down.

2. Avoid all high-impact sports and exercises.

3. Progress slowly and gradually. Avoid the temptation to do too much too soon.

4. Wear the right clothing. This should include good quality, appropriate footwear, so make sure to get good advice before you purchase.

5. Be aware of the climate when you exercise. If it is cold and you are outdoors, wrap up well. If it is warm make sure to wear breathable clothing. It is particularly important to avoid overheating, which is why the recommended exercises are gentler.

6. Drink plenty of fluids before, during and after your exercise.

7. Be in tune with your body. If you feel like you are challenging it, ease up immediately. Remember your aim is to have a baby and not to win an Olympic medal.

8. Include gentle stretching as part of your routine before and after you exercise.

RECOMMENDED EXERCISES

The best exercise for fertility is a combination of walking and gentle, meditative exercise such as the softer forms of yoga and chi gong. After this type of exercise you should feel peaceful and energised rather than tired. You might need to change how you understand fitness. If you are used to high sporting performance, the recommended exercises will seem quite tame, but remember to keep your eye on your new goal. You can return to higher intensity exercise a few months after you have had your baby.

Chi gong – My preferred exercise system is chi gong. Chi gong means 'energy work' and is a traditional Chinese healing exercise system, with principles similar to those of acupuncture. This exercise system includes tai chi as one of its forms and has been used for thousands of years to enhance health and fertility. Chi gong is the perfect exercise for fertility as it uses gentle movements, focused breathing and meditative techniques. All these deliver the benefit of stress reduction without taxing your body. A typical chi gong exercise program contains a series of movements that should take no more than fifteen minutes to perform. Ideally it should be performed in the morning upon waking and last thing at night before going to bed. You should perform chi gong in a warm environment where it is quiet and there is little distraction. Make sure it is in a place where you can stand, sit and lie comfortably. For many people this will be their bedroom. It is also a good idea to find a chi gong or tai chi class in your area. These classes are now easier to find all over the UK and Ireland. Try to find an instructor who is patient and who takes time to explain the system. It is very important not only to understand the physical movements, but also the breathing techniques and the mental aspect of the exercise.

The Fertility Code Chi Gong training system is also available on DVD or download from www.fertilitycode.com.

Walking – Walking is an excellent low-impact aerobic exercise that will help you lose weight. If you have done very little exercise before, try walking at low to moderate intensity for just ten or fifteen minutes and build up to your recommended duration per day. Walking is a simple and effective form of exercise and can be adjusted to any fitness level. Apart from a good pair of walking shoes or trainers you don't need any special equipment and it is a super exercise for aerobic fitness. It is also an exercise that can be performed throughout pregnancy as you are in total control of the intensity.

Yoga – There is some anecdotal evidence that yoga can increase fertility. Some studies have found that certain yoga postures can indeed increase blood flow to your reproductive organs, which may stimulate ovulation and make the uterus more ready for conception. Studies have found that couples who practice yoga alongside IVF treatment are more likely to conceive. This may be due to the relaxation aspects of yoga, such as meditation and breath work. There are many different forms of yoga and I recommend that you practice one of the gentler forms such as Hatha yoga and avoid the more intense forms such as Ashtanga or Bikram when you are trying to conceive.

Pregnant women can continue to practise yoga. You should take yoga classes designed specifically for pregnant women, however, and always with a qualified instructor. The instructor will modify the poses so that they are appropriate for pregnancy. There are some fertility yoga books available which can support your progress with this exercise system. *Yoga for Fertility Handbook* by Sue Dumais is a simple, easy to read book with great illustrations and detailed instructions. However, in practice it is difficult to learn yoga from a book and I think it is important that you find a good class and a teacher in your area who can lead you on the correct path.

Swimming – Swimming is another excellent exercise as long as it is performed gently. It is excellent for aerobic health and can also be helpful for losing weight if that is your goal. Because the water holds your body weight, this can be an excellent exercise for anyone with weak or sore joints, as there is no impact. For this reason it is also a good exercise for women who are pregnant, as it can help relieve stress and strain on muscles that are being stretched and challenged in pregnancy.

EXERCISE DURING PREGNANCY

Exercise is important for health, and pregnancy does not change this for most women. Exercise during pregnancy may help to shorten labour and birth, and it generally helps a woman to have a quicker recovery postpartum. More importantly it helps a woman to feel healthier during the pregnancy. There are a few things to watch out for when exercising while pregnant, however.

Watch your balance – After the first four months of pregnancy a woman's body will see changes that can alter her balance and it is easier to go off balance. Although the baby is very well protected by the amniotic sac if you were to fall, you should still be careful when exercising.

Stay off your back – Also after the fourth month of pregnancy, a woman's uterus will have grown out of her pelvis and the weight of it, when you are on your back, can depress the vena cava. This is the vein that carries deoxygenated blood from the upper half of the body to the heart. Depressing the vena cava reduces the amount of blood flow, and therefore oxygen, to the baby. Many women will find that they can become dizzy or light-headed if they lie on their backs. This is something that should always be avoided, not just during exercise. You should never lie on your back when exercising while pregnant, and even when you are resting you should lie on your side.

♀♂

CHAPTER SUMMARY

Exercise, when performed correctly, is very beneficial for fertility. It can help you to de-stress, enhance your emotional well-being and improve your sleep. Exercise can also play an important role in helping you manage your weight.

Attaining in or around your ideal weight can significantly improve your chances of conception, and once you have conceived, this will also help you to deliver a healthy baby.

In order to achieve your ideal weight, the Fertility Code Nutrition Plan plays a vital role. This plan is supported by exercise and you will perform less or more exercise depending on whether you need to lose or gain weight.

Follow a gradual approach, starting exercise slowly, without becoming exhausted. Increase the duration of your exercise until you reach the target appropriate for your weight control objective.

Maximise your comfort and safety. Be sure to wear good quality footwear and dress appropriately for the weather.

Exercise should always be low intensity and you should avoid overheating, making sure to hydrate properly before, during and after exercise.

♀ ♂

BMI CHART

▨ = Healthy weight

Height / Weight (lbs)	5'0"	5'1"	5'2"	5'3"	5'4"	5'5"	5'6"	5'7"
100	20	19	18	18	17	17	16	16
105	21	20	19	19	18	18	17	16
110	22	21	20	20	19	18	18	17
115	23	22	21	20	20	19	19	18
120	23	23	22	21	21	20	19	19
125	24	24	23	22	22	21	20	20
130	25	25	24	23	22	22	21	20
135	26	26	25	24	23	23	22	21
140	27	27	26	25	24	23	23	22
145	28	27	27	26	25	24	23	23
150	29	28	27	27	26	25	24	24
155	30	29	28	28	27	26	25	24
160	31	30	29	28	28	27	26	25
165	32	31	30	29	28	28	27	26
170	33	32	31	30	29	28	27	27
175	34	33	32	31	30	29	28	27
180	35	34	33	32	31	30	29	28
185	36	35	34	33	32	31	30	29
190	37	36	35	34	33	32	31	30
195	38	37	36	35	34	33	32	31
200	39	38	37	36	34	33	32	31
205	40	39	38	36	35	34	33	32
210	41	40	38	37	36	35	34	33
215	42	41	39	38	37	36	35	34
220	43	42	40	39	38	37	36	35
225	44	43	41	40	39	38	36	35
230	45	44	42	41	40	38	37	36
235	46	44	43	42	40	39	38	37
240	47	45	44	43	41	40	39	38
245	48	46	45	43	42	41	40	38
250	49	47	46	44	43	42	40	39
255	50	48	47	45	44	43	41	40
260	51	49	48	46	45	43	42	41
265	52	50	49	47	46	44	43	42
270	53	51	49	48	46	45	44	42

5'8"	5'9"	5'10"	5'11"	6'0"	6'1'	6'2"	6'3'	6'4"
15	15	14	14	14	13	13	13	12
16	16	15	15	14	14	14	13	13
17	16	16	15	15	15	14	14	13
18	17	17	16	16	15	15	14	14
18	18	17	17	16	16	15	15	15
19	18	18	17	17	17	16	16	15
20	19	19	18	18	17	17	16	16
21	20	19	19	18	18	17	17	16
21	21	20	20	19	19	18	18	17
22	21	21	20	20	19	19	18	18
23	22	22	21	20	20	19	19	18
24	23	22	22	21	20	20	19	19
24	24	23	22	22	21	21	20	20
25	24	24	23	22	22	21	21	20
26	25	24	24	23	22	22	21	21
27	26	25	24	24	23	23	22	21
27	27	26	25	24	24	23	23	22
28	27	27	26	25	24	24	23	23
29	28	27	27	26	25	24	24	23
30	29	28	27	27	26	25	24	24
30	30	29	28	27	26	26	25	24
31	30	29	29	28	27	26	26	25
32	31	30	29	29	28	27	26	26
33	32	31	30	29	28	28	27	26
34	33	32	31	30	29	28	28	27
34	33	32	31	31	30	29	28	27
35	34	33	32	31	30	30	29	28
36	35	34	33	32	31	30	29	29
37	36	35	34	33	32	31	30	29
37	36	35	34	33	32	32	31	30
38	37	36	35	34	33	32	31	30
39	38	37	36	35	34	33	32	31
40	38	37	36	35	34	33	33	32
40	39	38	37	36	35	34	33	32
41	40	39	38	37	36	35	34	33

Overcoming
Challenges

"When it is obvious that the goal is not being reached, don't adjust the goal, adjust the action steps"

Confucius

INTRODUCTION

By now you have gathered information and begun to take steps to ensure that you and your partner are in the best physical, mental and emotional health for conception. But for some couples it is inevitable that there will be more complex physical health issues that need to be addressed in order to increase your chances of having a baby.

During the initial consultation at the clinic we spend a lot of time going through the full health profile of our couples who are planning to have a baby. During this consultation process we leave no stone unturned in trying to identify any obstacles that might be in the way of achieving a successful pregnancy. We also recommend that our clients undergo a full fertility check with their GP, which will help to determine if there are any factors that might be having an impact on their fertility.

Almost 40 per cent of fertility issues relate to a female factor. A similar percentage relates to male issues and the rest are due to unexplained causes or multiple factors involving both partners. It is estimated that around 90 per cent of couples with infertility problems can be successfully treated. By following the Fertility Code you are already taking steps towards treating many of these issues. We will now look at some common fertility-related medical issues and treatment approaches.

ENDOMETRIOSIS

Endometriosis is probably the most common and also the most complex medical cause of fertility problems. It is estimated that around 15 per cent of women have this condition, but of those seeking assistance with fertility around 35 per cent will have it.

With endometriosis, the lining of the uterus – the endometrial tissue that sheds with each monthly period – begins to grow into other areas of the abdomen. These pieces of endometrium can grow anywhere in the pelvic area, including the ovaries, fallopian tubes, the bladder and the pelvic wall. This tissue responds to hormones, just as it would inside the uterus, except there is no way for it to exit the body as it should, and it can continue to grow. When it breaks down it can become inflamed and cause adhesions or scar tissue to form, as well as potentially causing blockages to the fallopian tubes.

If endometriosis becomes advanced and extensive, it can reduce a woman's chances of conception. It is not quite clear what causes endometriosis, but it does seem that there may be a genetic factor involved. It is also believed that weakness of the immune system may be a factor.

From a Chinese-medicine perspective endometriosis is frequently associated with a condition called blood stagnation or blood stasis syndrome. In Chinese medicine it is the qi (pronounced chi), or energy, that moves blood around your body, and it is the blood that nourishes that qi. Therefore if the blood isn't moving properly, it is because the qi isn't moving properly. Qi stagnates because of stress held within your body, or frequently because the blood itself isn't nourishing the qi. If you have endometriosis and you also have symptoms such as poor circulation, poor sleep, poor immunity, dry hair and skin, and brittle nails, then there is a strong chance that you have endometriosis due to blood stagnation caused initially by blood deficiency. Chinese medicine believes that this has three possible causes:

1. Genetics

2. Blood loss due to factors such as heavy periods, blood donation and accidents

3. Improper diet

Of these three causes, improper diet is the most common. Typically, it is not the food you eat that is the problem, but rather the food that you don't eat enough of. People who don't eat enough dark, leafy green vegetables will frequently have blood deficiency.

Whatever the cause, the solution to blood deficiency from a Chinese-medicine perspective is primarily based on nutrition and it is advised that you eat at least two portions of dark leafy green vegetables every day to improve this condition. The supplement spirulina, mentioned in the Fertility Code Nutrition Plan, is also an excellent blood tonic for this problem.

Western medical treatment of this condition sometimes includes birth control pills to regulate hormones but of course this isn't helpful if you are actively trying to conceive. In this case your GP may suggest laparoscopy surgery which involves the surgeon using a laser to remove the unwanted endometrial tissue. This is frequently very effective, depending on the location of the endometrial tissue and how extensive it is. Around half of women will conceive within eighteen months of having surgery.

ENDOMETRIOSIS

Definition	A condition in which endometrial tissue grows outside the uterus.
Potential symtoms	Painful menstrual periods, irregular or heavy bleeding, pain during intercourse.
Possible medical solutions	Laparoscopic surgery to remove the tissue and /or unblock tubes, and assisted conception treatments.
Success rates	Surgery: 40-60 per cent conceive within eighteen months of surgery. IVF: usual expected success rates.

POLYCYSTIC OVARY SYNDROME

Polycystic ovary syndrome (PCOS) is the most common ovulation disorder and the most common hormonal cause of fertility problems in women. About 10 per cent of women have PCOS.

In PCOS a hormonal dysfunction means that the ovaries are unable to produce one fully mature egg. Numerous follicles are stimulated but don't mature, and instead they form tiny cysts on the surface of the ovary. These cysts can exacerbate the condition by further disrupting hormonal secretions. The cysts can also produce male hormones, which can prevent ovulation occurring. Without creating the right hormonal environment, the possibility of ovulating a mature egg that is capable of being fertilised is diminished, and so are the chances of implantation.

Many women who have PCOS do ovulate, but they do so later in their cycle. When this happens the eggs may be of poorer quality and there can be an increased chance of miscarriage. For women who don't ovulate, medication to stimulate the process can help, but again the quality of the egg produced can be an issue.

The symptoms associated with PCOS include irregular periods, unwanted hair growth, acne and weight gain. Most women with PCOS have weight problems, with around half being seriously overweight. These are typical symptoms of PCOS, but quite often women with the condition will have no symptoms at all and it is only picked up with an ultrasound scan.

The causes of PCOS are not fully understood but recent evidence suggests that insulin sensitivity plays a significant role in the condition. When there are high levels of insulin present, this stimulates the ovaries and can cause excessive production of male hormones and anovulation (failure to ovulate).

Given the likely relationship with high insulin levels a possible solution to this would be to rebalance blood-sugar levels by eliminating refined carbohydrates and eating only slow-release carbohydrates that do not spike insulin levels, as recommended by the Fertility Code Nutrition Plan.

By addressing these dietary factors you are also likely to lose weight, and studies have shown that even a 10 per cent drop in body weight can produce normal ovulation in women with PCOS.

All aspects of the Fertility Code are very useful for women who have PCOS.

> ✤ The Fertility Code Nutrition Plan helps to achieve
> weight loss and helps to rebalance blood-sugar and

insulin levels.

- ✍ The Fertility Code exercise approach supports weight loss
- ✍ The Fertility Code Mind Programme deals with stress and helps to redress hormonal balance.

POLYCYSTIC OVARY SYNDROME	
Definition	Many small cysts are present on the ovaries. There are hormone imbalances and ovulation is irregular or absent.
Potential symtoms	Irregular periods, unwanted hair growth, acne and weight gain.
Possible medical solutions	Ovulation and follicle stimulating medications and IVF.
Success rates	Seventy per cent of those who take fertility medication ovulate, and of those, half will go on to conceive within six to nine months. A further 20 per cent conceive with assisted fertility treatments such as IVF.

BLOCKED FALLOPIAN TUBES

Blocked fallopian tubes are very common and account for approximately 20 per cent of female fertility problems. In order for a successful pregnancy to occur, the egg must travel through the fallopian tube to the uterus. If the tube is completely blocked, the sperm cannot reach the egg and conception cannot occur. Sometimes the tube is partially blocked, allowing the sperm to fertilise the egg. However, if the fertilised egg doesn't reach the uterus, an ectopic pregnancy occurs.

The most common reason for blocked fallopian tubes is that they have been intentionally blocked as a form of surgical contraception. It is possible to reverse this surgically.

A common unintentional cause of blocked fallopian tubes is tubal scar tissue. Fallopian tubes can become blocked when scar tissue forms inside and/or outside the tubes. The most common reason for the formation of scar tissue is infection. Conditions such as endometriosis and inflammatory bowel disease can cause scar tissue to form, which can close the fallopian tubes from either the inside or the outside.

Abdominal infections can also lead to fallopian tube blockage. This can arise following a ruptured appendix, gallbladder disease or any significant trauma that caused injury to the intestines. If a severe infection occurs in your body, your immune system responds to fight off the infection. One effect of this immune response can be the formation of scar tissue in and around the area affected. In these cases scar tissue in the pelvis can form across the outside of the fallopian tube or cause the end of the tube to close. The most common infection associated with fallopian tube blockage is pelvic inflammatory disease (PID). These infections are often, but not always, sexually transmitted and when they occur they can cause severe damage to any part of the tubes.

Blockage of the fallopian tubes can be difficult to detect because there are no symptoms. It is usually diagnosed using ultrasound or hysterosalpingogram (HSG) X-ray procedures, during which a dye is injected into the uterus and it is observed whether or not the dye travels through the tubes. If the dye stops in the tube or the tube swells, this indicates that there is a blockage.

The approach to correcting fallopian tube blockage in most cases will be to use an advanced laparoscopic surgical technique.

BLOCKED FALLOPIAN TUBES

Definition	Damaged, blocked or partially blocked fallopian tubes can prevent eggs from travelling to the uterus and sperm from getting to the egg. The main causes include pelvic inflammatory disease (PID), sexually transmitted diseases such as chlamydia, and surgery.
Potential symtoms	No symptoms.
Possible medical solutions	Laparoscopic surgery to open the tubes, if possible (where the blockage is small). Where surgery is not an option, or it fails, IVF is often recommended.
Success rates	Conception rates vary from as low as 10 per cent to as high as 70 per cent, depending on the severity of the blockage and the amount of scar tissue that develops after surgery.

♀♂

INFECTIONS

Untreated or undetected infections are frequently overlooked as a cause of fertility problems but it is thought that as much as 15 per cent of difficulties can be traced back to infections. Infections come from many sources. Some are sexually transmitted, such as chlamydia, genital herpes and syphilis. Some of these sexually transmitted diseases, such as chlamydia, can lie silently in your body, damaging your fertility without any symptoms or warning signs. There is also a host of other infections that are not sexually transmitted and can cause fertility difficulties, such as yeast infections like candida albicans.

Approximately 25 per cent of women seeking fertility treatment carry micro-organisms that may impair fertility. As well as causing difficulties with the female reproductive system these infections can harm and kill sperm. So if bacteria exist in the cervical mucus, they can attack the sperm and prevent it from penetrating the egg. The sperm itself can also carry bacteria from the man's body.

Many of these infections can be so subtle that they don't show any symptoms, which makes detection more difficult. The best way to detect infection in a woman's body is to get a cervical mucus test from your doctor.

If infection is detected both partners should be treated with antibiotics, because if both carry the infection and only one is treated they can soon be re-infected by their partner. In addition to antibiotics the Fertility Code Nutrition Plan and the recommended supplements will help to boost your immune system and prevent the recurrence of these infections.

IMMUNE SYSTEM FACTORS AND FERTILITY

A healthy immune system is important for your body to function normally. Your reproductive system, immune system and hormones are all interrelated. Anyone with a defective immune system will be more susceptible to diseases that can affect fertility. Experts believe that approximately 20 per cent of unexplained fertility problems relate to immune system disorders of some sort.

Women generally tend to have a stronger immune system than men and this is thought to be due to its reproductive role in protecting a foetus. There are immune cells that are involved with inflammatory response, and these cells play an essential role in the ovulation process. The immune cells are also involved in preparing the endometrium for implantation of a fertilised egg. Therefore, the healthier your immune system is, the less likely it is that your fertility will be compromised.

So if you are trying for a baby, being at your healthiest should improve your chances of conception and a healthy pregnancy. We know that even a short bout of flu or sickness can briefly affect sperm count and contribute towards ovulation irregularities.

We have witnessed many cases of long-term unexplained infertility that have been resolved when a couple has changed to a healthier lifestyle that strengthened their immune system. This includes every aspect of the Fertility Code: a nutritious diet, drinking enough water, stress reduction, appropriate exercise, adequate sleep and reducing toxins.

AUTOIMMUNE DISEASE AND FERTILITY

An autoimmune condition occurs when the immune system becomes faulty and turns on itself. This triggers inflammatory responses, which can harm healthy cells and tissue. There are many types of autoimmune diseases such as lupus, type 1 diabetes, Crohn's disease, multiple sclerosis and rheumatoid arthritis.

It is not known exactly why these immune system disorders occur, but there seems to be some genetic predisposition that acts together with environmental factors and perhaps viral infection.

Because women tend to have stronger immunity than men, autoimmune conditions are thought to affect women more often. Some autoimmune diseases may contribute to fertility problems in both sexes, whilst others do not hinder fertility at all. If you have an autoimmune disease, you should discuss it with your doctor or gynaecologist, who will advise you as to whether it is a factor in your fertility and recommend steps you can take to reduce the impact of that condition. This will involve assessing your medication, addressing specific triggers and improving your lifestyle and dietary issues. The Fertility Code can also help you to achieve much of this.

ANTIPHOSPHOLIPID SYNDROME

Antiphospholipid syndrome (APS) commonly combines with other autoimmune diseases, but can also present on its own. In APS antiphospholipid antibodies (a type of immune cell) interfere with the regular working of blood vessels, causing blood clotting. This syndrome can cause numerous pregnancy-related problems and may be responsible for fertility problems involving implantation failure.

Your GP or gynaecologist may order tests to determine if this autoimmune factor is an issue, and may prescribe a low dose of aspirin or other form of blood thinner as a preventative measure.

ANTI-SPERM ANTIBODIES

Both men and women can produce anti-sperm antibodies, although it is more common in men. Antibodies are normally produced in response to a foreign substance entering the body. In this case these antibodies are accidentally produced against sperm. When these antibodies attach to sperm cells, they hinder their movement and can make it much more difficult for them to pass through cervical mucus. The sperm cells can then clump together and be destroyed.

Men may develop these antibodies due to testicular injury or torsion (twisting of the testicle) or an infection. Men may also have antisperm antibodies for no apparent reason. It is not fully understood why women produce antisperm antibodies in their cervical mucus.

Tests can be conducted to see if this immune system disorder is affecting your chances of conception. If it is a factor, medications that suppress the immune system may be prescribed, and assisted reproductive technologies can also help to overcome this problem.

THYROID PROBLEMS

The hormone disruption that hypothyroidism (underactive thyroid) can cause may lead to irregular menstrual cycles, which can affect fertility. Both hypothyroidism and hyperthyroidism (overactive thyroid, or Graves' disease) are known to affect ovulation. Hypothyroidism can also cause cysts to form on the ovaries and can trigger an increased production of prolactin – the hormone that controls milk production in women who are not pregnant. Very high levels of prolactin may hamper ovulation.

Women who are hypothyroid are about four times more likely to miscarry than women who are not.

If your thyroid is an issue, the best thing you can do to enhance your fertility and minimise the risk of health complications is to seek treatment as soon as possible.

MISCARRIAGE

Many fertilised embryos, as many as half, fail to implant sufficiently for pregnancy to continue. Around 95 per cent of miscarriages occur in the first trimester of pregnancy and about 15 per cent of all pregnancies end in miscarriage.

When a miscarriage occurs during the first trimester of pregnancy, it is usually considered to be due to complications with the unborn baby. If a miscarriage happens after this time in the pregnancy it is usually considered to be due to an underlying health condition in the mother. It has to be said, however, that much is unknown about miscarriage and as many as 60 per cent are unexplained.

Reasons for miscarriage

Chromosome problems – Chromosomes are blocks of genetic code, or DNA. They contain a detailed set of instructions that determine a number of factors relating to the developing baby. An embryo is a union between sperm and egg and for a pregnancy to be successful the foetus needs to have forty-six chromosomes in total – twenty-three from the mother's egg and twenty-three from the father's sperm.

At the moment of conception something can go wrong and the foetus can receive too many or too few chromosomes. The reason why this happens is unclear, but it means that the foetus will not develop normally, resulting in a miscarriage. It is thought that up to two thirds of all early miscarriages are related to chromosome abnormalities.

Placental problems – The placenta links the mother's blood supply to her baby's. The hormone progesterone is produced to support the pregnancy in the first few weeks until the placenta has developed. If there isn't sufficient progesterone produced this can also lead to a miscarriage.

Autoimmune antibodies – Antibodies are produced by the

immune system when fighting infection. Women who have experienced recurrent miscarriages often have high levels of an antibody called antiphospholipid (aPL) in their blood. These antibodies can cause blood clots which can block the supply of blood to the foetus, which may result in a miscarriage. When there is a high level of aPL antibodies in the blood this is known as Hughes syndrome.

Problems with cervix and uterus structure – Problems and abnormalities with the uterus are more likely to lead to second trimester miscarriages. These structural problems can include fibroids, scarring on the surface of the uterus or a uterine septum, which is where a band of tissue runs down the middle of the uterus.

Sometimes the muscles at the neck of the uterus (the cervix) are too weak. This may have been caused by an injury in this area, or can have existed from birth. This weakness can cause the cervix to open too early during pregnancy, leading to a miscarriage. When this problem is identified, the treatment is a surgical stitch to close the cervix.

Risk factors

Although the reasons for miscarriage are not always known, there are several risk factors that increase the likelihood. Age is the most significant risk factor; miscarriage rates of 10 per cent for women under thirty rise to 20 per cent for women aged between thirty and forty. This rises to 50 per cent for women over forty-five. Of course there isn't anything you can do about your age but there are things you can do about the other risk factors that relate to you, such as:

- obesity
- smoking during pregnancy
- drug misuse during pregnancy (particularly cocaine)
- excessive intake of caffeine
- excessive alcohol intake

Of course by implementing the Fertility Code you will address all of these lifestyle-related risk factors.

ASSISTED REPRODUCTIVE TECHNOLOGIES

There are numerous medical fertility treatment options available to couples today. Some of you may have bought this book to help to prepare yourself for one of these treatment options. Or perhaps test results suggest that you should consider medical assistance and look to assisted reproductive technologies (ART) such as intrauterine insemination (IUI), in vitro fertilisation (IVF) or intracytoplasmic sperm injection (ICSI).

My work as an acupuncturist has led me to support many couples who receive ART treatments. Numerous studies have indicated that when acupuncture supports IVF treatment the success rates increase by almost 70 per cent.

The Fertility Code is excellent preparation for anyone considering IVF or other forms of ART. The approach to optimising fertility in preparation for unassisted conception is generally to make the couple as healthy as possible. The approach when trying to improve IVF outcomes is basically the same. You should focus on stress management and relaxation, optimal nutrition, detoxification, achieving your optimal weight and taking the appropriate amount of exercise.

There is considerable evidence that stress affects IVF outcomes, so the Fertility Code Mind Programme is particularly relevant, and you should learn and regularly practise the stress-management techniques we discussed in chapter two. Given that stress has an impact on fertility-related hormones and the fact that you will have considerable hormonal therapy during the IVF process, it is essential that you do everything you can to support yourself mentally and emotionally.

At my clinics I frequently bring clients through a three-month programmme that includes every element of the Fertility Code, supported by acupuncture. This enables couples to optimise their health both physically and mentally for the IVF journey. It is not uncommon for couples to find that during this preparation their vitality improves so much that they conceive prior to commencing their IVF treatment.

Intrauterine insemination (IUI)

Many couples who seek assisted reproductive technologies will try an intrauterine insemination (IUI) procedure. This is less invasive than in vitro fertilisation (IVF) and is performed as an outpatient procedure.

If you have been trying for several months, perhaps with the help of ovulation-stimulating medication, many specialists will recommend that a couple have an IUI procedure. Where the woman is under thirty-five the couple will often be encouraged to try for up to twelve months before seeking assistance. If she is over thirty-five an IUI may be considered after about six months.

The key factor in deciding whether a couple are candidates for IUI is having a proper understanding of what the fertility issue is. IUI works best when the woman can ovulate, either with the assistance of medication or not, and does not have an issue with her fallopian tubes. In cases of low sperm motility or poor sperm quality an IUI may also be considered, as the process of preparing the sperm for the IUI ensures that only better-quality sperm is used. The procedure itself places the sperm higher up in the uterus than would happen naturally and this makes the journey easier for the sperm.

Where the cause of a couple's infertility is unknown, an IUI will often be performed as a first-step in fertility treatments.

IUI procedure

The IUI procedure is straightforward, quick and relatively comfortable. Once the sperm has been collected and prepared, it is placed in a thin catheter about six inches long. The catheter is inserted into the vagina and the sperm is injected directly into the cervix or uterus. Once the catheter is removed, the cervix closes and prevents the sperm from coming back out. The entire process generally takes five minutes or less.

IUI variations

There are three main approaches for an IUI cycle.

Natural cycle – This is the basic IUI procedure. Here, insemination is planned for between days twelve and fifteen of the cycle and the woman's natural ovulation is used. Ovulation predictor kits may be used to indicate that ovulation is about to happen. Once the couple know that the woman is about to ovulate they go in to the clinic to complete the IUI process.

Medically-assisted cycle – Where a woman's ovulation is not happening regularly or when there isn't a strong enough hormone surge to support conception, fertility specialists may prescribe Clomid. This medication stimulates and produces stronger, more predictable ovulation. There are quite a few side effects of this medication, such as cramping, headache and mood swings. Post-ovulation ultrasounds are usually carried out to make sure that the ovaries have not been overstimulated.

Monitored cycle – Another approach taken by clinics is to observe the ovaries via ultrasound for a few days prior to when ovulation is expected. Once at least one mature follicle develops, the IUI is performed the next day. This is often supported by injecting human chorionic gonadotropin hormone (HCG) prior to the procedure to trigger full ovulation.

Success rates

Success rates of IUI procedures can vary a great deal. Most studies show conception rates to be somewhere between 10 and 20 per cent. This is just marginally higher than the chances of natural conception taking place; it is however seen as a valid first medically-assisted step in trying to conceive after self-timed natural attempts have failed.

Pros and cons of IUI

Like most assisted reproductive techniques, there are advantages and disadvantages to be considered when selecting IUI. If there is a blockage in the fallopian tubes, the IUI procedure cannot work. As there are no symptoms of fallopian tube blockage you could be spending time, money and effort when there is no possibility that it could work. When the woman has an irregular cycle, getting the correct timing of the IUI can also be challenging. In this case you will need to monitor for ovulation daily or else take medication to ensure timly ovulation.

One of the most significant benefits of IUI is that the sperm being used is washed and prepared prior to the process. This increases the viability of the sample. Since it is placed farther into the woman's body, low motility issues are also tackled.

IN VITRO FERTILISATION (IVF)

Fertility treatment approaches can be confusing for many couples. However, the more knowledge you have the less likely you are to feel apprehension. Fully understanding the IVF process can make a huge difference to how you feel about this treatment approach.

The IVF process

Ovarian stimulation

This first stage of IVF aims to produce at least eight follicles that will provide quality eggs for retrieval. Fertility drugs are used to stimulate the ovaries in a similar way to the natural process. However, because of their highly concentrated nature, the hormonal shots are capable of promoting the development of multiple follicles. This treatment can have side effects such as abdominal discomfort, breast tenderness and mood swings.

Egg retrieval

Before this step your doctor will monitor you to confirm that the follicles have matured. After administering anaesthesia, the doctor retrieves the eggs using a hollow needle guided by ultrasound into the ovary via the uterus. This procedure is called follicular aspiration. The eggs are then removed, rinsed and stored in an IVF incubator until they are ready for fertilisation.

Post-retrieval medication

After egg retrieval has taken place, the woman will frequently be given antibiotics to help prevent infection, sometimes steroids are also given if assisted hatching is part of the protocol. Progesterone might be used to help uterine lining development, and perhaps aspirin to prevent clotting in the tiny blood vessels that lead to the uterus. This should also improve blood flow to the reproductive organs.

Sperm retrieval

The man will provide a sperm sample. If there is a problem doing this the sperm may be removed surgically from the testicles. This will happen if there is no sperm in the ejaculate or if the man has had a vasectomy. The sperm is then washed and prepared for fertilisation.

Fertilisation and development of the embryo

After the sperm and egg have been retrieved, they will be combined into an embryo at the clinic. This is then placed in a special medium, containing protein, salt and antibiotics, and left in an incubator for a few days. The embryologist will regularly check the embryos and will perform the transfer when the embryo has developed adequately.

Embryo transfer

Prior to the transfer taking place, the clinic will perform some form of embryo screening. Frequently this will be done with five-day-old embryos, which are likely to have a better chance of implanting and growing into healthy babies.

The IVF process now moves to the embryo transfer stage. This does not usually require any medication and is done as an outpatient procedure. There is strong evidence that receiving acupuncture approximately thirty minutes prior to transfer, followed up by more acupuncture after transfer will increase your success rate by approximately 65 per cent. The embryos are suspended in fluid and placed in a catheter which is gently guided into the uterus and the embryos are placed on the womb lining. After the transfer, the woman is advised to take things easy for a day or two, and to avoid exercise and overheating. Remaining embryos may be frozen for use in the future.

The two-week wait

After embryo transfer comes the famous two-week wait. There is very little that can be done at this stage, except to take the prescribed progesterone and stay relaxed. We will frequently support our clients' relaxation during this time by performing one or two acupuncture treatments. After two weeks you can perform a pregnancy test, and if this is positive you are advised to confirm with a blood test for a completely accurate result.

Hopefully, this test will yield a positive result and your pregnancy will begin.

WHAT HAPPENS WHEN YOU FIND OUT YOU ARE PREGNANT?

Whether it comes from simply following the Fertility Code Programme or from medically assisted treatments supported by the programme, what happens now that you are pregnant? Well, first of all, congratulations! This is a profound moment, an amazing breakthrough for many couples, and you have every right to feel elated.

At this point you must take things easy and look after yourself as best you can. If you have had complications previously, book an appointment to see your doctor as soon as possible. They are likely to recommend an early scan at between six and eight weeks. Continue to follow the Fertility Code Nutrition Plan and take the supporting supplements. Continue to avoid caffeine, alcohol, tobacco, hot baths, saunas and steam rooms

Exercise at this stage should be minimal. Limit yourself to gentle strolls and easy chi gung exercises. Do not take any medications unless they have been prescribed by your doctor or obstetrician.

As you move from the first trimester into the second trimester any anxiety you might have in relation to the pregnancy should begin to fade. I would highly recommend that you continue with monthly acupuncture treatments for the duration of the pregnancy up until close to the day when your new baby arrives.

WHAT HAPPENS IF YOU FIND THAT YOU ARE NOT YET PREGNANT?

It is important to stay balanced and positive. See this as an opportunity to spend more time enhancing your health and fertility. Depending on the amount of time you have been trying to conceive naturally with the support of the Fertility Code, you may wish to book an appointment with your doctor to discuss what options are available to assist you.

CHAPTER SUMMARY

If you have implemented the Fertility Code Programme for a number of months and have not as yet successfully conceived there may be a physical and structural reason for this. In this case, you should consider having a full fertility check up with your doctor or obstetrician. As age is a factor I suggest following up on this after twelve months of trying to conceive if you are under thirty-five. If you are over thirty-five I recommend that you investigate sooner, after about four months.

- There are a variety of conditions that respond very well to medical interventions and once these have been addressed the Fertility Code will very often bring success within a few months.

- Implementing the Fertility Code is also helpful for couples who are seeking medical intervention to help with identified fertility problems.

- There are numerous assisted reproductive technologies available to couples today such as IUI, IVF and ICSI. The Fertility Code is excellent preparation for couples seeking such interventions and can dramatically increase success rates.

- When you become pregnant continue to implement the Fertility Code. At this time you must make sure to take the very best care of yourself and the Fertility Code Programme will ensure that you do just that.

Conclusion
Bringing it all together

"A journey of a thousand miles begins with a single step"

Laozi

I hope you now fully embrace the knowledge that you can take charge of your own fertility. You make the lifestyle choices that determine your diet, weight, exposure to toxins, exercise and even your thoughts and stress levels.

Whilst reading this book you will have been taking on board the overall message of the Fertility Code. Will following all steps of the Fertility Code guarantee that you will have a baby? Unfortunately not, but each step of the Fertility Code enhances your fertility as a couple. The more diligently you follow the Fertility Code the more improvements you should see to both you and your partner's health and fertility.

People come to my clinic for a variety of health reasons, but by far the main reason people come is to seek support in their quest to have a baby. When dealing with other medical complaints it is usually quite easy to determine if progress is being made. Simple questions like, *Does your back hurt less? Is your digestion better?* or, *Has your skin cleared?* are all usually quite easy to answer.

People coming to my clinic with the ultimate goal of having a baby will often only feel success has occurred when they are holding their newborn baby in their arms. Thankfully this happens often but there are also many checkpoints along the way, where you should be able to determine that the Fertility Code is working. I would recommend that you maintain a diary and track the improvements you feel are taking place with your general health as a consequence of following the Fertility Code.

For many people, implementing the Fertility Code will mean making significant lifestyle changes. Although these changes are worthwhile and you should soon witness the many benefits of making these adjustments, it is also understandable that this can be challenging. Implement the programme one step at a time, making daily adjustments until you feel that you are fully implementing the programme. Where should you start? Well I think that the following steps are vitally important for everyone:

- ♫ Nutrition is key – embrace the Fertility Code Nutrition Plan in its entirety.

- ♫ Determine your ideal body weight and move towards that target weight using proper nutrition and appropriate exercise.

- ♫ If you smoke, quit.

- ♫ Avoid coffee and all caffeine.

- ♫ Get the Fertility Code recommended supplements and start taking them.

- ♫ Improve stress management by attending classes and following the Fertility Code Mind Programme.

The key to succeeding with the Fertility Code is simply to take what you have learned from this book and put it into action. There are many exercises to perform and principles to implement. Take control of your fertility and create a sense of momentum as you work your way through the programme. Recognise that each step forward should bring you closer to your goal of having a healthy baby and building your family.

Following one aspect of the Fertility Code will be helpful, but it is through the combined effect of implementing all aspects of the programme that you will deliver the most profound outcomes in terms of your health and fertility. The Fertility Code Mind Programme will help you to properly manage any stress you are dealing with. Stress plays an influential role in the manner in which hormones work in your body. Good stress management is therefore very helpful to achieving healthy hormonal balance and studies indicate that this step alone will increase your fertility by as much as 60 per cent.

Following the Fertility Code Nutrition Plan and the recommended nutritional supplements will ensure that you have the optimum nutrients in your body when you achieve pregnancy. The nutrition and exercise plan will also help you to attain your optimum weight, a step that will smooth out your blood-sugar levels and improve your insulin sensitivity. The nutrition plan has a strong anti-inflammatory effect on your body. This and other aspects of the nutrition plan combine to promote healthy ovulation, and better quality and greater quantity of sperm, which improves conception rates and encourages the healthy development of your baby once you have conceived.

Implementing the Fertility Code Detox will reduce your exposure to toxins such as nicotine, alcohol and caffeine. There is strong evidence that people who avoid these toxins achieve a healthy pregnancy much quicker than those who do not. The advantages of not being exposed to such toxins will also accrue to your baby and undoubtedly benefit the long-term health of your child.

I have done my best to pass on the principles and tools that you can use to achieve significant improvements to your health and fertility. Whilst each part of the Fertility Code stands on its own merits, it is by bringing all these parts together that you bring a harmony to many diverse factors that influence your fertility. This puts you on the right road to a healthy pregnancy, a well developed baby and, once born, a lifetime of vibrant health for your child. These techniques have worked for me and for thousands of my clients.

As you work your way through this process and fully implement the Fertility Code, I want to make one small request. When you have achieved success, tell us about it. Share your success story so that it will inspire and motivate others on their own fertility journey. Please send your messages to dermot@fertilitycode.com.

Bringing a new life into the world is a wonderful gift and if you can give words of encouragement to others it can truly make a huge difference. Be part of the Fertility Code community and visit our website www.fertilitycode.com.

Until I hear from you, I would like to leave you with a famous Irish blessing:

May your God be with you and bless you,
May you see your children's children,
May you be poor in misfortunes and rich in blessings,
And may you know nothing but happiness from this day forward.

♀♂

Select Bibliography
and further reading

Attaman, J.A., Toth, T.L., Furtado, J., Campos, H., Hauser, R. and
Chavarro, J.E., 'Dietary Fat and Semen Quality Among Men
Attending a Fertility Clinic', *Human Reproduction* (2012) 27 (5):
1466–74.

Barbieri, R.L., Domar, A.D. and Loughlin, K.R., *Six Steps to Increased
Fertility*, Simon & Schuster, 2001.

Bari, M., Battista, N., Pirazzi, V. and Maccarrone, M., 'The Manifold
Actions of Endocannabinoids on Female and Male Reproductive
Events', *Frontiers in Bioscience* (2011) 2 (16): 498–516.

Blitzer, B., *The Infertility Workbook: A Mind-Body Program to Enhance
Fertility, Reduce Stress, and Maintain Emotional Balance*, New
Harbinger Publications, 2011.

Chavarro, J.E., Rich-Edwards, J.W., Rosner, B. and Willett, W.C.,
'A Prospective Study of Dairy Foods Intake and Anovulatory
Infertility', *Human Reproduction* (2007) 22 (5): 1340–7.

Chavarro, J.E., Wallet, W.C. and Skerrett, P., *The Fertility Diet:
Groundbreaking Research Reveals Natural Ways to Boost Ovulation and
Improve Your Chances of Getting Pregnant*, McGraw-Hill, 2007.

Cramner, D.W., Xu, H. and Sahi, T., 'Adult Hypolactasia, Milk
Consumption, and Age-Specific Fertility', *American Journal of
Epidemiology* (1994) 139 (3): 282–9.

Domar, A.D., Clapp, D., Slawsby, E.A., Dusek, J., Kessel, B. and
Freizinger, M., 'Impact of Group Psychological Interventions on
Pregnancy Rates in Infertile Women', *Fertility and Sterility* (2000)
73 (4): 805–11.

Domar, A.D., Rooney, K.L, Wiegand, B., Orav, E.J., Alper, M.M.,
Berger, B.M. and Nikolovski, J., 'Impact of a Group Mind/Body
Intervention on Pregnancy Rates in IVF Patients', *Fertility and
Sterility* (2011) 95 (7): 2269–73.

Dooley, M., *Fit for Fertility*, Hodder Mobius, 2007.

Ebbesen, S.M., Zachariae, R., Mehlsen, M.Y., Thomsen, D., Højgaard, A., Ottosen, L., Petersen, T. and Ingerslev, H.J., 'Stressful Life Events Are Associated with a Poor In-Vitro Fertilization (IVF) Outcome: A Prospective Study', *Human Reproduction* (2009) 24 (9): 2173–82.

Forges, T., Monnier-Barbarino, P., Alberto, J.M., Guéant-Rodriguez, R.M., Daval, J.L. and Guéant, J.L., 'Impact of Folate and Homocysteine Metabolism on Human Reproductive Health', *Human Reproduction* (2007) 13 (3): 225–38.

Ganmaa, D. and Sato, A., 'The Possible Role of Female Sex Hormones in Milk from Pregnant Cows in the Development of Breast, Ovarian and Corpus Uteri Cancers', *Medical Hypotheses* (2005) 65 (6): 1028–37.

Giudice, L.C., 'Infertility and the Environment: The Medical Context', *Seminars in Reproductive Medicine* (2006) 24 (3): 129–33.

Glenville, M., *Getting Pregnant Faster*, Kyle Cathie, 2008.

Hauser, R., Meeker, J.D., Duty, S., Silva, M.J. and Calafat, A.M., 'Altered Semen Quality in Relation to Urinary Concentrations of Phthalate Monoester and Oxidative Metabolites', *Epidemiology* (2006) 17: 682–91.

Hugo, S., *The Fertile Body Method: A Practitioner's Manual: The Applications of Hypnosis and Other Mind-Body Approaches for Fertility*, Crown House Publishing, 2009.

Jensen, T.K., Hjollund, N.H.I., Brink Henriksen, T., Scheike, T., Kolstad, H., Giwercman, A., Ernst, E., Bonde, J.P., Skakkebæk, N.E. and Olsen, J., 'Does Moderate Alcohol Consumption Affect Fertility?', *British Medical Journal* (1998) 317: 505.

Malekinejad, H., Scherpenisse, P. and Bergwerff, A.A. 'Naturally Occurring Estrogens in Processed Milk and in Raw Milk (From Gestated Cows)', *Journal of Agricultural and Food Chemistry* (2006) 54 (26): 9785–91.

Mendola, P., Messer, L.C. and Rappazzo, K. 'Science Linking Environmental Contaminant Exposures with Fertility and Reproductive Health Impacts in the Adult Female', *Fertility and Sterility* (2008) 89 (2 Supplement): e81–94.

Saldeen, P. and Saldeen, T. 'Women and Omega-3 Fatty Acids', *Obstetrical and Gynecological Survey* (2004) 59 (10): 722–30.

Silva, P.D., Cool, J.L. and Olson, K.L. 'Impact of Lifestyle Choices on Female Infertility', *Journal of Reproductive Medicine* (1999) 44 (3): 288–96.

Taylor, C., 'Calcium in Oocyte Maturation: Calcium Signals and Human Oocyte Activation: Implications for Assisted Conception', *Human Reproduction* (1994) 9 (6): 980–4.

Unfer, V., Casini, M.L., Costabile, L., Mignosa, M., Gerli, S. and Di Renzo, G.C., 'Endometrial Effects of Long-Term Treatment with Phytoestrogens: A Randomized, Double-Blind, Placebo-Controlled Study', *Fertility and Sterility* (2004) 82 (1): 145–8.

Van der Steeg, J.W., Steures, P., Eijkemans, M.J.C., Habbema, J.D.F., Hompes, P.G.A., Burggraaff, J.M., Oosterhuis, G.J.E., Bossuyt, P.M.M., Van der Veen, F. and Mol, B.W.J., 'Obesity Affects Spontaneous Pregnancy Chances in Subfertile, Ovulatory Women', *Human Reproduction* (2008) 23 (2): 324–8.

Whitcomb, B.W., Bodach, S.D., Mumford, S.L., Perkins, N.J., Trevisan, M., Wactawski-Wende, J., Liu, A. and Schisterman, E.F., 'Ovarian Function and Cigarette Smoking', *Paediatric and Perinatal Epidemiology* (2010) 24 (5): 433–40.

Wilcox, A., Dunson, D. and Baird, D., 'The Timing of the "Fertile Window" in the Menstrual Cycle: Day Specific Estimates from a Prospective Study', *British Medical Journal* (2000) 321: 1259–62.

Quinn, T. and Heller, B., *Infertility Cleanse: Detox, Diet and Dharma for Fertility*, Findhorn Press, 2011.

DERMOT O'CONNOR

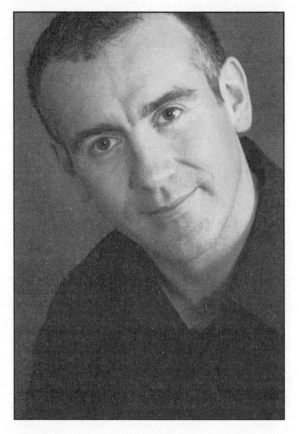

If you would like a personal consultation with Dermot O'Connor, or to take part in one of his workshops in the UK or Ireland, please contact:
E-mail: dermot@fertilitycode.com
Tel: +44 (0) 871 218 0300 (UK) or +353 (0) 1 667 2222 (Ireland)